T0273780

Small Animal Oncology

Editors

CRAIG A. CLIFFORD
PHILIP J. BERGMAN

VETERINARY CLINICS OF NORTH AMERICA: SMALL ANIMAL PRACTICE

www.vetsmall.theclinics.com

May 2024 • Volume 54 • Number 3

ELSEVIER

1600 John F. Kennedy Boulevard • Suite 1800 • Philadelphia, Pennsylvania, 19103-2899
http://www.vetsmall.theclinics.com

**VETERINARY CLINICS OF NORTH AMERICA: SMALL ANIMAL PRACTICE Volume 54, Number 3
May 2024 ISSN 0195-5616, ISBN-13: 978-0-443-13059-5**

Editor: Stacy Eastman
Developmental Editor: Varun Gopal

Veterinary Clinics of North America: Small Animal Practice (ISSN 0195-5616) is published bimonthly by Elsevier Inc., 360 Park Avenue South, New York, NY 10010-1710. Months of issue are January, March, May, July, September, and November. Business and Editorial Offices: 1600 John F. Kennedy Blvd., Ste. 1800, Philadelphia, PA 19103-2899. Customer Service Office: 3251 Riverport Lane, Maryland Heights, MO 63043. Periodicals postage paid at New York, NY and additional mailing offices. Subscription prices are $391.00 per year (domestic individuals), $100.00 per year (domestic students/residents), $503.00 per year (Canadian individuals), $544.00 per year (international individuals), $100.00 per year (Canadian students/residents), and $220.00 per year (international students/residents). For institutional access pricing please contact Customer Service via the contact information below. To receive student/resident rate, orders must be accompanied by name of affiliated institution, date of term, and the *signature* of program/residency coordinator on institution letterhead. Orders will be billed at individual rate until proof of status is received. Foreign air speed delivery is included in all *Clinics* subscription prices. All prices are subject to change without notice. **POSTMASTER:** Send address changes to *Veterinary Clinics of North America: Small Animal Practice*, Elsevier Health Sciences Division, Subscription Customer Service, 3251 Riverport Lane, Maryland Heights, MO 63043. Customer Service (orders, claims, online, change of address): Elsevier Periodicals Customer Service, Elsevier Health Sciences Division Subscription **Customer Service 3251 Riverport Lane Maryland Heights, MO 63043. Tel: 1-800-654-2452 (U.S. and Canada); 314-447-8871 (outside U.S. and Canada). Fax: 314-447-8029. E-mail: journalscustomerservice-usa@elsevier.com (for print support); journalsonlinesupport-usa@elsevier.com (for online support).**

Reprints. For copies of 100 or more of articles in this publication, please contact the Commercial Reprints Department, Elsevier Inc., 360 Park Avenue South, New York, NY 10010-1710. Tel.: 212-633-3874; Fax: 212-633-3820; E-mail: reprints@elsevier.com.

Veterinary Clinics of North America: Small Animal Practice is also published in Japanese by Inter Zoo Publishing Co., Ltd., Aoyama Crystal-Bldg 5F, 3-5-12 Kitaaoyama, Minato-ku, Tokyo 107-0061, Japan.

Veterinary Clinics of North America: Small Animal Practice is covered in *Current Contents/Agriculture, Biology and Environmental Sciences, Science Citation Index, ASCA, MEDLINE/PubMed (Index Medicus), Excerpta Medica,* and *BIOSIS.*

Contributors

EDITORS

CRAIG A. CLIFFORD, DVM, MS
Diplomate of the American College of Veterinary Internal Medicine; Oncology, Medical Oncologist, BluePearl Pet Hospital - Malvern, Malvern, Pennsylvania, USA

PHILIP J. BERGMAN, DVM, MS, PhD
Director, Clinical Studies, Diplomate of the American College of Veterinary Internal Medicine; Oncology, Director, Clinical Studies, Veterinary Centers of America, Oncologist, Katonah Bedford Veterinary Center, Bedford Hills, New York, USA; Adjunct Associate Faculty, Memorial Sloan Kettering Cancer Center, New York, New York, USA

AUTHORS

PHILIP J. BERGMAN, DVM, MS, PhD
Director, Clinical Studies, Diplomate of the American College of Veterinary Internal Medicine; Oncology, Director, Clinical Studies, Veterinary Centers of America, Oncologist, Katonah Bedford Veterinary Center, Bedford Hills, New York, USA; Adjunct Associate Faculty, Memorial Sloan Kettering Cancer Center, New York, New York, USA

JEFFREY N. BRYAN, DVM, MS, PhD
Diplomate of the American College of Veterinary Internal Medicine (Oncology); Professor of Veterinary Oncology, Comparative Oncology Radiobiology and Epigenetics Laboratory, Professor of Oncology, University of Missouri Columbia, Ellis Fischel Cancer Center, Columbia, Missouri, USA

ESTHER CHON, DVM
Diplomate of the American College of Veterinary Internal Medicine (Oncology); Head of Veterinary Affairs, Vidium Animal Health, Scottsdale, Arizona, USA

CRAIG A. CLIFFORD, DVM, MS
Diplomate of the American College of Veterinary Internal Medicine; Oncology, Medical Oncologist, BluePearl Pet Hospital - Malvern, Malvern, Pennsylvania, USA

WILLIAM T.N. CULP, MD
Diplomate of the American College of Veterinary Surgeons; Professor, Small Animal Surgery, ACVS Founding Fellow of Surgical Oncology, ACVS Founding Fellow of Minimally Invasive Surgery, ACVS Founding Fellow of Oral and Maxillofacial Surgery, Professor, University of California-Davis, School of Veterinary Medicine, Davis, California, USA

ANDI FLORY, DVM
Diplomate of the American College of Veterinary Internal Medicine (Oncology); Chief Medical Officer, PetDx, Encinitas, California, USA

TRACY L. GIEGER, DVM
Clinical Professor, Department of Clinical Sciences, College of Veterinary Medicine, North Carolina State University, Raleigh, North Carolina, USA

DAVID HAWORTH, DVM, PhD
President, Vidium Animal Health, Scottsdale, Arizona, USA

WILLIAM HENDRICKS, PhD
Chief Scientific Officer, Vidium Animal Health, Scottsdale, Arizona, USA

CHAD M. JOHANNES, DVM
Diplomate of the American College of Internal Medicine (SAIM, Oncology); Associate Professor, Colorado State University, Fort Collins, Colorado, USA

JULIUS M. LIPTAK, BVSc, MVetClinStud, FANZCVSc
Diplomate of the American College of Veterinary Surgery – Small Animal; Diplomate European College of Veterinary Surgeons; ACVS Founding Fellow, Surgical Oncology, ACVS Founding Fellow, Oral and Maxillofacial Surgery, RCVS Specialist in Surgical Oncology, Capital City Specialty & Emergency Animal Hospital, Kanata, Ontario, Canada

CHRISTINE MULLIN, VMD
Diplomate of the American College of Internal Medicine (Oncology); Oncologist, BluePearl Pet Hospital - Malvern, Malvern, Pennsylvania, USA

MICHAEL W. NOLAN, DVM, PhD
Professor, Department of Clinical Sciences, College of Veterinary Medicine, North Carolina State University, Raleigh, North Carolina, USA

GERALD POST, DVM
Diplomate of the American College of Veterinary Internal Medicine (Oncology); Chief Veterinary Officer, OneHealthCompany, Inc, Palo Alto, California, USA

LUCAS RODRIGUES, DVM, PhD
Head of Veterinary Research, OneHealthCompany, Inc, Palo Alto, California, USA

BERNARD SÉGUIN, DVM, MS
Diplomate of the American College of Veterinary Surgeons; ACVS Founding Fellow, Surgical Oncology, ACVS Founding Fellow, Oral and Maxillofacial Surgery, Central Victoria Veterinary Hospital, Victoria, British Columbia, Canada

KAI-BIU SHIU, BVMS, MRCVS
DACVIM (Oncology); Medical Oncologist, VCA VESVSC, Middleton, Wisconsin, USA

DOUGLAS H. THAMM, VMD
Diplomate American College of Veterinary Internal Medicine (Oncology); Barbara Cox Anthony Professor of Oncology, Flint Animal Cancer Center, College of Veterinary Medicine and Biomedical Sciences, Colorado State University, Fort Collins, Colorado, USA

KRISTEN WEISHAAR, DVM, MS
DACVIM (Oncology); Veterinary Oncologist, Colorado State University Flint Animal Cancer Center, CSU Veterinary Teaching Hospital, Fort Collins, Colorado, USA

MICHELLE WHITE, DVM, PhD
Head of Science, OneHealthCompany, Inc, Palo Alto, California, USA

HEATHER WILSON-ROBLES, DVM
Diplomate of the American College of Veterinary Internal Medicine (Oncology); Chief Medical Officer, Volition Veterinary Diagnostic Development, Henderson, Nevada, USA; Clinician Scientist, Ethos Discovery, Washington DC, USA; Staff Veterinarian, The Oncology Service, United Veterinary Health, Springfield, Virginia, USA

ZACHARY M. WRIGHT, DVM
DACVIM (Oncology); Medical Director, VCA Animal Diagnostic Clinic, Dallas, Texas, USA

Contents

focused on the use of locoregional therapies and stenting of malignant obstructions. Although significant assessment of veterinary IO techniques is
still necessary, early evaluation of these varying techniques is demonstrating promising results.

Precision medicine focuses on the clinical management of the individual
patient, not on population-based findings. Successes from human precision medicine inform veterinary oncology. Early evidence of success for
canines shows how precision medicine can be integrated into practice.
Decreasing genomic profiling costs will allow increased utilization and
subsequent improvement of knowledge base from which to make better
informed decisions. Utility of precision medicine in canine oncology will
only increase for improved cancer characterization, enhanced therapy selection, and overall more successful management of canine cancer. As
such, practitioners are called to interpret and leverage precision medicine
reports for their patients.

Clinical care of osteosarcoma (OSA) in dogs has seen little change during
the past 2 decades, relying on amputation and platinum-based chemotherapy for pain control and survival. Recent advancements offer hope
for improved outcomes. Genomic research reveals shared genetic abnormalities between canine and human OSA. Multidimensional imaging provides valuable staging and prognostic information. Limb-sparing
approaches including stereotactic body radiation therapy are routine.
Ablative therapies such as microwave ablation and histotripsy show promise. Immunotherapy including cell therapy and immune checkpoint inhibition are available. Radiopharmaceuticals are tuned to target OSA cells
directly. These innovations may enhance treatment and prognosis for
dogs with OSA.

The past decade has seen incredible advances in blood-based cancer detection in people and in dogs - yet this represents only a glimpse of the
benefits these tests can provide to patients. The clinical uses of this technology range from screening asymptomatic individuals for early detection
to use as an aid in diagnosis when cancer is suspected, to cancer monitoring both during and after treatment. This article summarizes the benefits of
early cancer detection and examines use cases and methods of blood-
based cancer detection in dogs, including quantitative, qualitative, and alternative approaches.

Stereotactic radiotherapy (SRT) involves the precise delivery of highly conformal, dose-intense radiation to well-demarcated tumors. Special equipment and expertise are needed, and a unique biological mechanism distinguishes SRT from other forms of external beam radiotherapy. Families find the convenient schedules and minimal acute toxicity of SRT appealing. Common indications in veterinary oncology include nasal, brain, and bone tumors. Many other solid tumors can also be treated, including spinal, oral, lung, heart-base, liver, adrenal, and prostatic malignancies. Accessibility of SRT is improving, and new data are constantly emerging to define parameters for appropriate case selection, radiation dose prescription, and long-term follow-up.

New knowledge and data can influence the treatment options of dogs and cats affected by neoplasms. Partial limb amputation with the use of a prosthesis is possible in dogs. Newer studies attempt to define better and understand the complications and limb function associated with this approach. Limb sparing is an alternative to amputation, and three-dimensional printing allows the manufacturing of personalized endoprostheses. Finally, the recommended approach for the excision of cutaneous mast cell tumors (MCTs) is with proportional margins. In dogs, grade shifting might have occurred when removing a recurrent MCT or soft tissue sarcoma.

This article explains the authors' experiences about opportunities, perspectives, and considerations required to initiate clinical studies in a veterinary oncology practice. These details include the infrastructure required for appropriate study training for all staff. Negotiation of scope of work and fees for service with study sponsors is also discussed. Finally, although generally similar, the article also describes management of clinical studies in academic and private practice settings.

VETERINARY CLINICS OF NORTH AMERICA: SMALL ANIMAL PRACTICE

SERIES OF RELATED INTEREST

Veterinary Clinics: Exotic Animal Practice
https://www.vetexotic.theclinics.com/
Advances in Small Animal Care
https://www.advancesinsmallanimalcare.com/

THE CLINICS ARE NOW AVAILABLE ONLINE!
Access your subscription at:
www.theclinics.com

Preface

Advancements in Veterinary Oncology

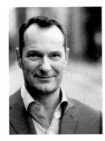 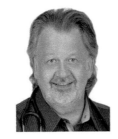

Craig A. Clifford, DVM, MS   Philip J. Bergman, DVM, PhD

Editors

We are entering an exciting time in veterinary oncology, whereby the seeds sowed within the comparative oncology realm many years ago are now coming to bloom in the form of a greater molecular understanding of cancer in companion animals. The comparative animal model has garnered significant interest in both industry and academia. The ensuing research has yielded breakthrough discoveries, from advanced diagnostics to novel therapies, which provide opportunities to improve our patients' longevity and quality of life.

This issue of *Veterinary Clinics of North America: Small Animal Practice* highlights our field's wide breadth of advancements, with diverse topics ranging from new drugs for mast cell tumors, chemotherapy-induced diarrhea, and lymphoma, updates in the field of interventional radiology, updates on stereotactic radiation, the use of liquid biopsy, the role of clinical trials in veterinary oncology, understanding veterinary precision-based medicine, a review of current and future immunotherapeutics, and updates from the field of surgical oncology.

Vet Clin Small Anim 54 (2024) xi–xii
https://doi.org/10.1016/j.cvsm.2023.12.001
0195-5616/24/© 2023 Published by Elsevier Inc.

We hope the reader will share our outlook—that the future of veterinary oncology is bright.

Craig A. Clifford, DVM, MS
BluePearl Malvern
40 three tun road
Malvern, PA 19355, USA

Philip J. Bergman, DVM, PhD
Clinical Studies
Veterinary Centers of America
Katonah-Bedford Veterinary Center
546 North Bedford Road
Bedford Hills, NY 10507, USA

Memorial Sloan Kettering Cancer Center
New York, NY 10065, USA

E-mail addresses:
Cliffdoc2000@yahoo.com (C.A. Clifford)
Philip.Bergman@VCA.com (P.J. Bergman)

Cancer Immunotherapy

Philip J. Bergman, DVM, MS, PhD[a,b,c,*]

KEYWORDS

- Cancer • Immunotherapy • Cancer vaccine • Monoclonal antibody • Canine
- Feline

KEY POINTS

- The immune system is generally divided into **2 primary components**: the *innate immune response* and the highly specific but more slowly developing *adaptive or acquired immune response*.
- Immune responses can be further separated by whether they are induced by exposure to a foreign antigen (an "active" response) or if they are transferred through serum or lymphocytes from an immunized individual (a "passive" response).
- The ideal cancer immunotherapy agent should be able to discriminate between cancer and normal cells (ie, specificity), be potent enough to kill a small or large numbers of tumor cells (ie, sensitivity), and lastly, be able to prevent the recurrence of the tumor (ie, durability).
- Tumor immunology and immunotherapy is one of the most exciting and rapidly expanding fields, with cancer immunotherapy now recognized as one of the pillars of treatment alongside surgery, radiation, and chemotherapy.

INTRODUCTION

The term "immunity" is derived from the Latin word *immunitas*, which refers to the legal protection afforded to Roman senators holding office. While the immune system is normally thought of as providing protection against infectious disease, the immune system's ability to recognize and eliminate cancer is the fundamental rationale for the immunotherapy of cancer. Multiple lines of evidence support a role for the immune system in managing cancer, including (1) spontaneous remissions in cancer patients without treatment; (2) the presence of tumor-specific cytotoxic T-cells within tumor or draining lymph nodes; (3) the presence of monocytic, lymphocytic, and plasmacytic cellular infiltrates in tumors; (4) the increased incidence of some types of cancer in immunosuppressed patients; and (5) documentation of cancer remissions with the use of immunomodulators.[1–3] With molecular biology tools and a greater understanding of mechanisms to harness the immune system, effective tumor immunotherapy is now a reality. This new class of therapeutics offers a more targeted and therefore precise

a Clinical Studies, VCA; b Katonah Bedford Veterinary Center, Bedford Hills, NY, USA;
c Memorial Sloan-Kettering Cancer Center, New York, NY, USA
* Katonah Bedford Veterinary Center, Bedford Hills, NY.
E-mail address: philip.bergman@vca.com

Vet Clin Small Anim 54 (2024) 441–468
https://doi.org/10.1016/j.cvsm.2023.12.002   vetsmall.theclinics.com

approach to the treatment of cancer. Cancer immunotherapy is now recognized as one of the pillars of treatment alongside surgery, radiation, and chemotherapy.

Tumor Immunology

Cellular components

The immune system is generally divided into 2 *primary components*: the *innate immune response* and the highly specific but more slowly developing *adaptive or acquired immune response*. Innate immunity is rapidly acting but typically not very specific and includes physico-chemical barriers (eg, skin and mucosa); blood proteins such as complement, phagocytic cells (macrophages, neutrophils, dendritic cells [DCs], and natural killer [NK] cells); and cytokines which coordinate and regulate the cells involved in innate immunity. Adaptive immunity is thought of as the acquired arm of immunity that allows for exquisite specificity, an ability to remember the previous existence of the pathogen (ie, "memory"), differentiate self from non-self, and, importantly, the ability to respond more vigorously upon repeat exposure to the pathogen. Adaptive immunity consists of T and B lymphocytes. The T cells are further divided into CD8 (cluster of differentiation) and MHC (major histocompatibility complex) class I cytotoxic helper T cells (CD4 & MHC class II), memory T cells, and regulatory T cells (Treg). B lymphocytes produce antibodies (humoral system) which may activate complement, enhance phagocytosis of opsonized target cells, and induce antibody-dependent cellular cytotoxicity. B-cell responses to tumors are thought by many investigators to be less important than the development of T-cell mediated immunity. Still, there is little evidence to support this notion fully.[4] The innate and adaptive arms of immunity are not mutually exclusive; they are linked by (1) the innate response's ability to stimulate and influence the nature of the adaptive response and (2) the sharing of effector mechanisms between innate and adaptive immune responses.

Immune responses can be further separated by whether they are induced by exposure to a foreign antigen (an "active" response) or if they are transferred through serum or lymphocytes from an immunized individual (a "passive" response). While both approaches can be extremely specific for an antigen of interest, one important difference is the inability of passive approaches to generally confer memory. The principal components of the active/adaptive immune system are lymphocytes, antigen-presenting cells, and effector cells. Furthermore, responses can be subdivided by whether they are specific for a certain antigen or a nonspecific response, whereby immunity is attempted to be conferred by upregulating the immune system without a specific target. These definitions are helpful as they allow methodologies to be more completely characterized, such as active-specific, passive-nonspecific, and so forth.

Immune surveillance

The idea that the immune system may actively prevent the development of neoplasia is termed "cancer immunosurveillance." Sound scientific evidence supports some aspects of this hypothesis[5–8] including (1) interferon (IFN)-γ protects mice against the growth of tumors, (2) mice lacking IFN-γ receptor were more sensitive to chemically induced sarcomas than normal mice and were more likely to develop tumors spontaneously, (3) mice lacking major components of the adaptive immune response (T and B cells) have a high rate of spontaneous tumors, and (4) mice that lack IFN-γ and B/T cells develop tumors, especially at a young age.

Immune evasion by tumors

There are significant barriers to the generation of effective antitumor immunity by the host. Many tumors evade surveillance mechanisms and grow in immunocompetent hosts as easily illustrated by the overwhelming numbers of people and animals succumbing to cancer. There are multiple ways in which tumors evade the immune response including (1) immunosuppressive cytokine production (eg, transforming growth factor-beta [TGF-β] and interleukin (IL)-10),[9,10] (2) impaired DC function via inactivation ("anergy") and/or poor DC maturation through changes in IL-6/IL-10/vascular endothelial growth factor/granulocyte-macrophage colony–stimulating factor (GM-CSF),[11] (3) induction of Treg, which were initially called suppressor T cells (CD4/CD25/CTLA-4/GITR/Foxp3 positive cells which can suppress tumor-specific CD4/CD8+ T cells),[12] (4) MHC I loss through structural defects, changes in B2-microglobulin synthesis, defects in transporter-associated antigen processing or actual MHC I gene loss (ie allelic or locus loss), and (5) MHC I antigen presentation loss through B7-1 attenuation (B7-1 is an important co-stimulatory molecule for CD28 mediated T-cell receptor and MHC engagement) when the MHC system in #4 remains intact.

Nonspecific Tumor Immunotherapy

Dr William Coley, a New York surgeon in the early 1900s, noted that some cancer patients developing incidental bacterial infections survived longer than those without infection.[13] Coley developed a bacterial "vaccine" (killed cultures of *Serratia marcescens* and *Streptococcus pyogenes* known as "Coley's toxins") to treat people with sarcomas which provided complete response rates of approximately 15%. Unfortunately, high failure rates and significant side effects lead to discontinuation of this approach. His seminal work laid the foundation for nonspecific modulation of the immune response in the treatment of cancer. There are numerous nonspecific tumor immunotherapy approaches ranging from biological response modifiers (BRMs) to recombinant cytokines as discussed in the following sections.

Biological response modifiers

BRMs are molecules that can modify the biological response of cells to changes in their external environment, which in the context of cancer immunotherapy could easily span nonspecific and specific immunotherapies. This section will be discussing nonspecific BRMs (sometimes termed "immunopotentiators") which are often related to bacteria and/or viruses.

One of the earliest BRM discoveries after Coley's toxin was the use of bacillus Calmette-Guérin (BCG; interestingly, Guérin was a veterinarian). BCG is the live attenuated strain of *Mycobacterium bovis,* and intravesical instillation in the urinary bladder causes a significant local inflammatory response which results in antitumor responses.[14] The use of BCG in veterinary patients was first reported by Owen and Bostock in 1974 and has been investigated with numerous types of cancers including urinary bladder carcinoma, osteosarcoma (OSA), lymphoma, prostatic carcinoma, transmissible venereal tumor, mammary tumors, sarcoids, squamous cell carcinoma, and others.[2,3,15–17] LDI-100, a product containing BCG and human chorionic gonadotropin, was compared to vinblastine in dogs with measurable grade II or III mast cell tumors.[18] Response rates were 28.6% and 11.7%, respectively, and the LDI-100 group had significantly less neutropenia. It is particularly exciting for the field of veterinary cancer immunotherapy to potentially be able to use a BRM product which has greater efficacy and less toxicity than a chemotherapy standard of care. Unfortunately, LDI-100 is not commercially available at present.

Corynebacterium parvum is another BRM which has been investigated for a number of tumors in veterinary medicine including melanoma and mammary carcinoma.[19,20] Other bacterially derived BRMs include attenuated *Salmonella typhimurium* (VNP20009), mycobacterial cell wall deoxyribonucleic acid (DNA) complexes (abstracts only at present), and bacterial superantigens.[21,22] Mycobacterial cell walls contain muramyl dipeptide (MDP) which can activate monocytes and tissue macrophages. Muramyl tripeptide-phosphatidylethanolamine (MTP-PE) is an analog of MDP. When encapsulated in multilamellar liposomes (L-MTP-PE), monocytes and macrophages uptake MTP leading to activation and subsequent tumoricidal effects through induction of multiple cytokines, including IL–1a, IL-1b, IL-7, IL-8, IL-12, and tumor necrosis factor.[23] L-MTP-PE has been investigated in numerous tumors in human and veterinary patients, including OSA, hemangiosarcoma, and mammary carcinoma.[23–27] Another mycobacterial cell wall fraction agent called Immunocidin received US Department of Agriculture (USDA) approval for intralesional use in canine mammary gland tumors. This product was also recently investigated with intravenous use and adjuvant doxorubicin in dogs with splenic hemangiosarcoma, but no prolongation in survival was noted compared to historical outcomes with adjuvant doxorubicin alone.[28]

Oncolytic viruses have also been used as nonspecific anticancer BRMs in human and veterinary patients.[29] Adenoviruses have been engineered to transcriptionally target canine OSA cells and have been tested in vitro and in normal dogs with no major signs of virus-associated side effects.[30–32] Similarly, canine distemper virus (CDV), the canine equivalent of human measles virus, has been used in vitro to infect canine lymphocyte cell lines and neoplastic lymphocytes from dogs with B and T cell lymphoma,[33] with high infectivity rates, suggesting that CDV may be investigated in the future for the treatment of dogs with lymphoma.

Imiquimod (Aldara) is a novel BRM that is a toll-like receptor 7 agonist.[34] Imiquimod has been reported as a successful treatment for Bowen's disease (multicentric squamous cell carcinoma in situ) and other skin diseases in humans. Twelve cats with Bowen's-like disease were treated topically with imiquimod 5% cream and initial and all subsequent new lesions responded in all cats.[35] An additional cat (with pinnal actinic keratoses and squamous cell carcinoma) and dog with cutaneous melanocytomas have subsequently been reported to have been successfully treated with topical imiquimod 5% cream.[36,37] It, therefore, appears that imiquimod 5% cream is well tolerated, and further studies are warranted to further examine its usefulness in cats and dogs with other skin tumors that are not treatable through standardized means.

Recombinant cytokines, growth factors, and hormones

A number of investigations using recombinant cytokines, growth factors, or hormones in various fashions for human and veterinary cancer patients have been reported to date. Many have investigated the in vitro and/or in vivo effects of the soluble cytokine (eg, IFNs, IL-2, IL-12, IL-15, and so forth with or without suicide gene therapy),[38–53] liposome encapsulation of the cytokine (eg, liposomal IL-2),[39,54–57] or use of a virus, cell, liposome-DNA complex, plasmid, or other mechanism to express or downregulate the cytokine (eg, recombinant poxvirus expressing IL-2).[54,58–66] The European Committee for Medicinal Products for Veterinary Use adopted a positive opinion in March, 2013 for the veterinary product Oncept IL-2 (feline poxvirus expressing recombinant feline IL-2). This product also received conditional licensure from the USDA Center for Veterinary Biologics (CVB) in 2015, but this conditional licensure lapsed in 2020 and the product is no longer commercially available in North America.

Specific Tumor Immunotherapy

Overview

The ultimate goal for a tumor immunotherapy with a specific target is elicitation of an antitumor immune response which results in clinical regression of a tumor and/or its metastases. There are numerous types of specific tumor immunotherapies in phase

I to III trials across a wide range of tumor types. Responses to cancer vaccines and other cancer immunotherapies may take several months or more to appear due to the slower speed of induction of the adaptive arm of the immune system as outlined in **Table 1**. This has necessitated the development of an alternative and more immunotherapeutic-based response system for human studies and this is highly likely necessary in the future for veterinary studies.[67] The ideal cancer immunotherapy agent would be able to discriminate between cancer and normal cells (ie, specificity), be potent enough to kill a small or large numbers of tumor cells (ie, sensitivity), and lastly, be able to prevent the recurrence of the tumor (ie, durability).

The immune system detects tumors through specific tumor-associated antigens (TAAs) and/or abnormal disease-associated antigens (DAAs) that are potentially recognized by both CTLs and antibodies.[68–71] TAAs and/or DAAs may be common to a particular tumor type, be unique to an individual tumor, or may arise from mutated gene products such as ras, p53, p21, and/or others. While unique TAAs may be more immunogenic than the other aforementioned shared tumor antigens, they are not practical targets because of their narrow specificity. Most shared tumor antigens are normal cellular antigens that are overexpressed in tumors. The first group to be identified was termed cancer testes antigens due to expression in normal testes, but they are also found in melanomas and various other solid tumors such as the MAGE/BAGE gene family. This article will highlight those approaches which appear to hold particular promise in human clinical trials and many which have been tested to date in veterinary medicine.

A variety of approaches have been taken to date to focus the immune system on the aforementioned targets, including (1) whole cell, tumor cell lysate, and/or subunit vaccines (autologous or made from a patient's own tumor tissue; allogeneic or made from individuals within a species bearing the same type of cancer; or whole cell vaccines from γ-irradiated tumor cell lines with or without immunostimulatory cytokines),[60,72–88] (2) vaccines which immunize with syngeneic and/or xenogeneic (different species than recipient) plasmid DNA (or other strategies) designed to elicit antigen-specific humoral and cellular immunity[89–104] (to be discussed in more detail later in this article), (3) viral, viruslike nanoparticle, and/or viral vector-based methodologies designed to be oncolytic and/or deliver genes encoding TAAs, telomerase, and/or immunostimulatory cytokines,[105–119] (4) DC or CD40-activated B-cell vaccines (which are commonly loaded or transfected with TAAs, DNA or ribonucleic acid from TAAs, or tumor lysates)[120–129] and adoptive cell transfer (the "transfer" of specific populations of immune effector cells in order to generate a more powerful and focused antitumor immune response; to be discussed in more detail later in this article with clinically relevant recent advances).[130–132]

There has been a remarkable expansion of companies offering autologous cancer vaccines for the treatment of cancer in a variety of veterinary species. Much of that expansion is due to limited regulatory oversight of autologous products due to the Virus-Serum-Toxin Act instituted in 1913. While these products are typically considered safe, there are extremely limited data around efficacy.[133–135] The USDA-CVB has increased regulatory scrutiny of these products starting in 2017 with Veterinary Services Memorandum (VSM) #800.121. In 2020, the USDA-CVB also increased regulatory scrutiny on conducting safety and efficacy studies for non-autologous cancer immunotherapeutics with VSM #800.126.

Antibody-based therapies

Antibody (Ab) approaches for cancer immunotherapy include monoclonal antibodies (mAbs),[136–139] anti-idiotype Abs (an idiotype is an immunoglobulin sequence unique to each B lymphocyte, and therefore Abs directed against these idiotypes are referred

Table 1
Comparison of chemotherapy and various antitumor immunotherapies

Treatment Type	Mechanism of Action	Tumor-Associated Aantigens or Target-Dependent	Specificity	Sensitivity	Response Time	Durability of Response
Chemotherapy	Cytotoxicity	No	Poor	Variable	Hours–days	Variable
Antitumor vaccine	Immune response	Yes	Good	Good	Weeks–months	Variable–long
Monoclonal antibodies	Immune response	Yes	Good	Good	Weeks	Variable
Checkpoint inhibitors	Immune response	No	Low	Moderate	Weeks–months	Long

to as anti-idiotype),[140] conjugated Abs (antibody conjugated to a toxin, chemotherapy, radionuclide, and so forth),[141] and engineered Ab "variants"[142,143] such as bispecific mAbs (can bind to 2 different targets at the same time), single-chain variable fragments (often used as artificial T-cell receptors), single-chain Abs, and so forth.

Rituximab (anti-human CD20 mAb; Rituxan, Biogen & Genentech, Inc.) was the first mAb approved by the Food and Drug Administration (FDA)[144] in 1997 and as of August 2023, there are over 100 FDA-approved mAbs for the treatment of various human cancers. In those 25+ years, a remarkably greater understanding of protein-engineering techniques, reciprocation between the immune system and cancer cells, as well as mechanisms of action and resistance for mAbs have allowed for therapeutic Ab development to explode.[143,145]

Based on the significant improvement in remission and survival length of human patients with B-cell non-Hodgkin's lymphoma (NHL) treated with rituximab and standard of care multiagent chemotherapy (and the lack of rituximab binding to canine CD20), numerous groups in veterinary medicine are in pursuit of similar caninized or felinized anti-CD20 mAb approaches.[146-154] Particular initial excitement and promise was noted in early pilot studies with caninized anti-CD20 and CD-52 mAbs (Vet Therapeutics, San Diego, CA, USA then purchased by Aratana, Inc.) for canine B-cell and T-cell NHL, respectively. In 2015 and 2016, each product (Blontress and Tactress, respectively) received USDA-CVB licensure, but subsequent unpublished studies did not show target binding or improvement in clinical outcomes compared to standard of care chemotherapy.[155] Based on rituximab's remarkable track record and continually expanding list of indications (within the previously envisioned area of B-cell neoplasia but now outside of oncology in the treatment of non-oncologic B-cell disorders), this author looks ardently forward to the clinical development of 1E4 (and other anti-CD19/20/21 mAbs) as well as other mAb targets for dogs, cats, and other veterinary species afflicted with cancer and other diseases.[156-161]

Cancer vaccines

One particularly exciting vaccine approach targets HER-2 with an attenuated listeria therapeutic vaccine or a DNA vaccine approach.[96,162,163] The listeria methodology was utilized by Mason and colleagues in dogs with appendicular OSA after being treated with amputation and adjuvant carboplatin chemotherapy.[164] The results from this phase I study are particularly exciting as it translated into a median survival time approaching 3 years. It is currently unknown how much of the therapeutic efficacy is from the xenogeneic human HER-2 versus the listeria. This lyophilized product from Aratana ("AT-014") received USDA-CVB conditional licensure in early 2018 and was further evaluated with a multicenter clinical safety study to potentially move the product to full licensure. Unfortunately, vaccine-origin listeria abscesses were noted in a handful of dogs.[165,166] This zoonotic threat precipitated the removal of this commercially available product in 2020. The original liquid version of this product was utilized in a COTC trial (COTC026) and the results have not been published to date.

This author developed a xenogeneic DNA vaccine program for melanoma in collaboration with human investigators from Memorial Sloan-Kettering Cancer Center.[167,168] Preclinical and clinical studies by our laboratory and others have shown that xenogeneic DNA vaccination with tyrosinase family members (eg, tyrosinase, GP100, GP75, others) can produce immune responses resulting in tumor rejection or protection and prolongation of survival while syngeneic vaccination with orthologous DNA does not induce immune responses. While tyrosinase may not appear to be a preferred target in amelanotic canine melanoma due to poor expression when assessed by immunohistochemistry (IHC),[169] more appropriate/sensitive polymerase chain reaction (PCR)–based studies and other IHC-based studies document significant tyrosinase overexpression in melanotic and amelanotic melanomas across species.[170–175] These studies provided the impetus for the development of a xenogeneic tyrosinase (or similar melanosomal glycoproteins) DNA vaccine program in canine malignant melanoma (CMM). Cohorts of dogs received increasing doses of xenogeneic plasmid DNA encoding either human tyrosinase (huTyr), murine GP75 (muGP75), murine tyrosinase (muTyr), muTyr ± HuGM-CSF (both administered as plasmid DNA), or muTyr "off-study" intramuscularly biweekly for a total of 4 vaccinations. We and collaborators have investigated the antibody and T-cell responses in dogs vaccinated with huTyr. Antigen-specific (huTyr) IFN-γ T-cells were found along with 2-fold to 5-fold increases in circulating antibodies to huTyr which can cross react to canine tyrosinase, suggesting the breaking of tolerance.[176,177] The clinical results with prolongation in survival have been reported previously.[167,168] The results of these trials demonstrate that xenogeneic DNA vaccination in CMM (1) is safe, (2) leads to the development of anti-tyrosinase antibodies and T cells, (3) is potentially therapeutic, and (4) is an attractive candidate for further evaluation in an adjuvant, minimal residual disease phase II setting for CMM. Based on these studies a multi-institutional safety and efficacy trial for USDA licensure in dogs with locally controlled stage II/III oral melanoma was initiated in 2006 with granting of conditional licensure in 2007, which represented the first US governmental regulatory agency approval of a vaccine to treat cancer across species. Results of this licensure trial documented a statistically significant improvement in survival for vaccinates versus controls and a full licensure for the huTyr-based canine melanoma vaccine from USDA-CVB was received in December 2009 (Oncept, Merial, Inc.).[178] Recently, other investigators have reported safety and feasibility results of a pilot study in 6 dogs with melanoma given huTyr plasmid DNA (ie, similar to Oncept), but instead of the typical needle-free transdermal delivery, a novel tattoolike "micro-seeding" delivery system was utilized.[179]

Kaser-Hotz and colleagues reported on concurrent use of Oncept and external beam radiation as many dogs with oral malignant melanoma may not be able to undergo surgery for local tumor control.[180] This pilot study determined that concurrent use was well tolerated with no unexpected toxicities. Ottnod and colleagues[181] performed a single-site retrospective study on 30 dogs with stage II to III oral malignant melanoma (15 each with and without use of Oncept). They determined that those dogs receiving Oncept did not achieve a greater progression-free survival, disease-free interval, or median survival time than dogs that did not receive the vaccine. Contrary to the aforementioned prospective USDA 5-site licensure trial,[178] this study had less than 35% of cases treated surgically with margins 1 mm or more, suggesting a significant lack of local tumor control. Furthermore, contrary to the aforementioned prospective USDA 5-site licensure trial, the Ottnod and colleagues study, similar to other noncontrolled retrospective studies, either had a wide variety of other treatments utilized in both the nonvaccinate and vaccinate groups, had small numbers of patients investigated, and/or the cause (in the context of local or distant disease) of death and/or progression of disease was not reported.[182–185] This author reported at the 2016 VCS meeting the outcomes of 320 dogs with malignant melanoma treated with Oncept across VCA oncology centers. The long-term median outcomes noted in that study are extremely similar to those we reported from the USDA 5-site prospective licensure trial and compare highly favorably to outcomes reported with standardized therapies without Oncept. Not surprisingly, the smaller poorly controlled retrospective studies do not appear to mirror the results seen in larger and more highly controlled studies.

Human clinical trials utilizing various xenogeneic melanosomal antigens as DNA (or peptide with adjuvant) vaccination began in 2005.[186-189] To further highlight xenogeneic DNA vaccination as a platform to target other possible antigens for other histologies, we have completed a phase I trial of murine CD20 for dogs with B-cell lymphoma (USDA-CVB conditionally licensed it as Canine Lymphoma Vaccine from Merial Inc. (now Boerhinger-Ingelheim Animal Health). This conditional licensure lapsed in 2020 and is no longer commercially available. We have also investigated the efficacy of local tumor control and use of xenogeneic DNA vaccination in dogs with digit malignant melanoma.[190] These investigations led to the development of a canine digit melanoma staging scheme and found an improvement in survival compared to historical outcomes with digit amputation only. We also documented a decreased prognosis for dogs with advanced stage disease and/or increased time from digit amputation to the start of vaccination. Phillips and co-investigators[170] have also reported the overexpression of tyrosinase in equine melanoma, determined the safety and optimal use of the needle-free delivery device into the pectoral region with Oncept, and documented antigen-specific humoral responses after vaccination in all horses.[191] Oncept also appears to be safe for use in cats and in a penguin case report.[192,193]

A small subset of dogs with malignant melanoma have exon 11 KIT gene mutations,[194,195] and therefore the more routine use of KIT testing by PCR of CMM and subsequent use of c-kit small-molecule inhibitors (particularly in dogs with advanced stage disease and/or lack of response to Oncept) should be considered. Furthermore, with somatic mutations in NRAS and PTEN being found in CMM[196] similar to human melanoma hotspot sites, these may represent logical drugable targets in the future.

The Future of Cancer Immunotherapy

Tumor immunology and immunotherapy is one of the most exciting and rapidly expanding fields at present. Significant resources are focused on mechanisms to simultaneously stimulate an antitumor immune response while minimizing the immunosuppressive aspects of the tumor microenvironment. Similar resources are also focused on ways to stimulate the "abscopal effect" which is derived from the Latin "ab" (position away from) and "scopus" (mark or target). The abscopal effect is when 1 tumor is treated locally and it causes other tumors outside the local treatment area to regress, presumably through immune-based mechanisms.[197] While this was hypothesized with radiation by RH Mole in 1953, the appreciation for this has exploded recently with cancer immunotherapeutics.

The recent elucidation and blockade of immunosuppressive cytokines (eg, TGF-β, IL-10 and IL-13) and/or the negative costimulatory molecule CTLA-4[198,199] and PD-1 (programmed cell death 1 or CD279),[200] along with the functional characterization of myeloid derived suppressor cells and T regulatory cells,[7,201-204] have dramatically improved cell-mediated immunity to tumors by "taking the brake" off the immune system. Immunotherapy is unlikely to become a sole modality in the treatment of cancer as the traditional modalities of surgery, radiation, and/or chemotherapy are extremely likely to be used in combination with immunotherapy in the future. Like any form of anticancer treatment, immunotherapy appears to work best in a minimal residual disease setting, suggesting its most appropriate use will be in an adjuvant setting with local tumor therapies such as surgery and/or radiation.[205] Similarly, the long-held belief that chemotherapy (non-corticosteroid) attenuates immune responses from cancer vaccines is beginning to be disproven through investigations on a variety of levels.[206-209]

The aforementioned greatly expanded molecular understanding of the immune system has recently translated into human cancer immunotherapeutics which confer a survival benefit such as the use of the checkpoint inhibitor anti-CTLA-4 Ab, ipilimumab (Yervoy, Bristol-Myers Squibb), and the selective BRAF inhibitors, vemurafenib (Zelboraf, Genetech) and dabrafenib (GSK2118436, GlaxoSmithKline), in patients who are BRAF V600 mutation positive. Currently, FDA-approved Abs directed against another checkpoint inhibitor known as PD-1 receptor or against human PDL-1 (L = ligand) such as nivolumab (Opdivo, Bristol-Myers Squibb), pembrolizumab (Keytruda, Merck), and others have generated the most excitement due to ~ 20% to 30% of human patients having durable objective tumor responses.[200,210] The highest objective tumor response rates have been seen to date in patients treated with concurrent PD-1 and CTLA-4 checkpoint inhibitors.[210–212] Furthermore, pembrolizumab was given FDA approval for unresectable or metastatic, microsatellite instability-high (MSI-H) or mismatch repair deficient (dMMR) solid tumors that have progressed following prior treatment.[213] This is truly revolutionary as it represents the first cancer-agnostic FDA approval and is one of the many recent FDA approvals based on single-arm studies. There are currently over 100 different checkpoint inhibitors in development and the immuno-oncology (IO) "pendulum" has swung from the previous primarily target-dependent approaches to the current checkpoint inhibitor target-independent approach. The IO pendulum over time is highly likely to come back to the middle with a concurrent target-dependent approach (ie, vaccine or similar) alongside target-independent checkpoint inhibitors.[214,215]

Very few biomarkers of response with these clinically important agents have been found to date unfortunately, except for fecal microbiome perturbations and tumors which generate numerous neoantigens from tumor-specific mutations.[216–218] This further highlights why pembrolizumab was given FDA approval for MSI-H or dMMR solid tumors as these tumors "throw off" comparatively much higher numbers of neoantigens. A highly innovative personalized human cancer vaccine taking advantage of this biomarker-based approach utilizes the neoantigens specific to that individual's cancer, as they are not present in normal tissues and are highly immunogenic.[219]

Another area of extreme promise in IO is adoptive cell therapy/transfer (ACT).[220] One type of ACT is CAR-T (chimeric antigen receptor-T cells). Other cell types can be utilized with CAR; for example, if using NK cells, then this would be termed CAR-NK. The cells are harvested from a patient and then genetically engineered to express a CAR on their cell surface with expansion in vitro before being reinfused back into the patient.[221] This CAR is specifically designed to recognize a specific TAA with a domain responsible for activating the T-cell when the CAR-T binds its TAA. The latest generations of CAR-T are engineered to contain important costimulatory domains that further enhance the immune response against the cancer cell containing the TAA. In 2017, an expert panel of the FDA called ODAC (Oncologic Drugs Advisory Committee) unanimously (10–0) recommended approval of CTL019 (tisagenlecleucel), an investigational CAR-T therapy utilizing CD19 as its CAR of choice for patients with B-cell acute lymphoblastic leukemia. Many CAR-T studies have found greater than 80% to 90% objective tumor responses, but side effects, including death can occur and relapses, can be frequent.[221,222] Furthermore, CAR-Ts are currently difficult to make and carry a high cost of goods to produce, making for a treacherous, but not impossible, commercial development path in veterinary medicine. One intriguing approach to reduce costs is to use an allogeneic CAR, especially CAR-NK, but significant logistical hurdles are also ahead due to activity and possible immunogenicity concerns.[223]

An additional form of ACT that has garnered significant interest in veterinary oncology utilizes an autologous patient tumor-based vaccination strategy followed by apheresis and ex-vivo T-cell expansion, which is then infused back into the patient with IL-2. This program is from Elias Animal Health and is called Elias Cancer Immunotherapy (ECI). In a pilot study of 14 dogs with appendicular OSA, ECI was performed after limb amputation.[224] The side effects were considered mild and typically grade 1 or 2. The median disease-free interval was 213 days with a median survival of 415 days and 5 dogs survived greater than 2 years. These pilot data are extremely exciting as it appears to be superior to historical outcomes with adjuvant carboplatin.[225–229] At this time (August 2023), we are eagerly awaiting the results of a larger USDA licensure trial in dogs with OSA treated with limb amputation followed by randomization to carboplatin versus ECI.

Checkpoints, checkpoint inhibitors, and other adoptive cell transfer technologies like CAR-T and others are also starting to be better understood and pursued in veterinary diseases.[130,230–274] Furthermore, the exciting race to develop commercial veterinary specific IO therapeutics like checkpoint inhibitors and CAR-T is currently ongoing with a handful of animal health companies. At the time of writing (August 2023), we anticipate in late 2023 the commercial release of gilvetmab, a caninized anti-PD-1 USDA conditionally licensed monoclonal antibody from Merck Animal Health. As these therapeutics reduce immune tolerance and more easily generate specific antitumor immune responses in patients, pathologic autoimmunity was predicted and is now being seen clinically in human patients as a side effect.[211,275,276]

An intriguing new area of IO utilizes high-intensity focused ultrasound (HIFU) or other hyperthermia modalities. These trigger the release of damage-associated molecular patterns and improve immune cell infiltration into tumors with an increase in NK and CD8+ T cells. Early results in mice and people suggest improved response rates with HIFU and checkpoint inhibitors compared to either alone, similar to radiation and checkpoint inhibitors.[250,277–279] This highly likely goes beyond simply turning an IO "cold" tumor into an IO "hot" tumor and the aforementioned neo-epitope creation by these modalities. This author ardently looks forward to further HIFU and combinatorial study strategies in veterinary oncology.[280–284]

In summary, the future looks extremely bright for immunotherapy. Similarly, the veterinary oncology profession is uniquely able to greatly contribute to the many advances to come in this field. Unfortunately, what works in a mouse will often not reflect the outcome in human cancer patients. Therefore, comparative immunotherapy studies utilizing veterinary patients may be able to better "bridge" murine and human studies. To this end, a large number of cancers in dogs and cats appear to be remarkably stronger models for counterpart human tumors than presently available murine model systems.[196,285–295] This is likely due to a variety of reasons including, but not limited to, extreme similarities in the biology of the tumors (eg, chemoresistance, radioresistance, sharing metastatic phenotypes and site selectivity, and so forth), spontaneous syngeneic cancer (vs typically an induced and/or xenogeneic cancer in murine models), and finally that the dogs and cats that are spontaneously developing these tumors are outbred, immune-competent, and live in the same environment that humans do. This author ardently looks forward to the time when cancer immunotherapy plays the same significant role in the treatment and/or prevention of cancers in veterinary patients like it currently does in human cancers.

DISCLOSURE

Dr P.J. Bergman is a co-inventor on patent US7556805B2 and was the veterinary principal investigator for the canine melanoma vaccine Oncept which received USDA-CVB conditional licensure in 2007 and full licensure in December of 2009. He also receives a minority royalty stream payment.

REFERENCES

1. Rosenberg SA. Karnofsky memorial lecture: The immunotherapy and gene therapy of cancer. J Clin Oncol 1992;10(2):180–99.
2. Theilen GH, Hills D. Comparative aspects of cancer immunotherapy: immunologic methods used for treatment of spontaneous cancer in animals. J Am Vet Med Assoc 1982;181:1134–41.
3. MacEwen EG. An immunologic approach to the treatment of cancer. Vet Clin N Am 1977;7:65–75.
4. Reilly RT, Emens LA, Jaffee EM. Humoral and cellular immune responses: independent forces or collaborators in the fight against cancer? Curr Opin Invest Drugs 2001;2:133–5.
5. Smyth MJ, Godfrey DI, Trapani JA. A fresh look at tumor immunosurveillance and immunotherapy. Nat Immunol 2001;2:293–9.
6. Wallace ME, Smyth MJ. The role of natural killer cells in tumor control–effectors and regulators of adaptive immunity. Springer Semin Immunopathol 2005;27: 49–64.
7. Itoh H, Horiuchi Y, Nagasaki T, et al. Evaluation of immunological status in tumor-bearing dogs. Vet Immunol Immunopathol 2009;132:85–90.
8. Schmiedt CW, Grimes JA, Holzman G, et al. Incidence and risk factors for development of malignant neoplasia after feline renal transplantation and cyclosporine-based immunosuppression. Vet Comp Oncol 2009;7:45–53.
9. Catchpole B, Gould SM, Kellett-Gregory LM, et al. Immunosuppressive cytokines in the regional lymph node of a dog suffering from oral malignant melanoma. J Small Anim Pract 2002;43:464–7.
10. Zagury D, Gallo RC. Anti-cytokine Ab immune therapy: present status and perspectives. Drug Discov Today 2004;9:72–81.
11. Morse MA, Mosca PJ, Clay TM, et al. Dendritic cell maturation in active immunotherapy strategies. Expet Opin Biol Ther 2002;2:35–43.
12. Yamaguchi T, Sakaguchi S. Regulatory T cells in immune surveillance and treatment of cancer. Semin Cancer Biol 2006;16:115–23.
13. Carlson RD, Flickinger JC Jr, Snook AE. Talkin' Toxins: From Coley's to Modern Cancer Immunotherapy. Toxins 2020;12.
14. Herr HW, Morales A. History of bacillus Calmette-Guerin and bladder cancer: an immunotherapy success story. J Urol 2008;179:53–6.
15. Owen LN, Bostock DE. Proceedings: Tumour therapy in dogs using B.C.G. Br J Cancer 1974;29:95.
16. MacEwen EG. Approaches to cancer therapy using biological response modifiers. Vet Clin North Am Small Anim Pract 1985;15:667–88.
17. Klein WR, Rutten VP, Steerenberg PA, et al. The present status of BCG treatment in the veterinary practice. In Vivo 1991;5:605–8.
18. Henry CJ, Downing S, Rosenthal RC, et al. Evaluation of a novel immunomodulator composed of human chorionic gonadotropin and bacillus Calmette-Guerin for treatment of canine mast cell tumors in clinically affected dogs. Am J Vet Res 2007;68:1246–51.
19. Parodi AL, Misdorp W, Mialot JP, et al. Intratumoral BCG and Corynebacterium parvum therapy of canine mammary tumours before radical mastectomy. Cancer Immunol Immunother 1983;15:172–7.
20. MacEwen EG, Patnaik AK, Harvey HJ, et al. Canine Oral Melanoma: Comparison of Surgery Versus Surgery Plus Corynebacterium parvum. Cancer Invest 1986;4(5):397–402.

21. Thamm DH, Kurzman ID, King I, et al. Systemic administration of an attenuated, tumor-targeting Salmonella typhimurium to dogs with spontaneous neoplasia: phase I evaluation. Clin Cancer Res 2005;11:4827–34.

22. Dow SW, Elmslie RE, Willson AP, et al. In vivo tumor transfection with superantigen plus cytokine genes induces tumor regression and prolongs survival in dogs with malignant melanoma. J Clin Invest 1998;101:2406–14.

23. Kleinerman ES, Jia S-F, Griffin J, et al. Phase II study of liposomal muramyl tripeptide in osteosarcoma: The cytokine cascade and monocyte activation following administration. J Clin Oncol 1992;10:1310–6.

24. MacEwen EG, Kurzman ID, Vail DM, et al. Adjuvant therapy for melanoma in dogs: results of randomized clinical trials using surgery, liposome-encapsulated muramyl tripeptide, and granulocyte macrophage colony-stimulating factor. Clin Cancer Res 1999;5:4249–58.

25. Teske E, Rutteman GR, vd Ingh TS, et al. Liposome-encapsulated muramyl tripeptide phosphatidylethanolamine (L-MTP-PE): a randomized clinical trial in dogs with mammary carcinoma. Anticancer Res 1998;18:1015–9.

26. Kurzman ID, MacEwen EG, Rosenthal RC, et al. Adjuvant therapy for osteosarcoma in dogs: results of randomized clinical trials using combined liposome-encapsulated muramyl tripeptide and cisplatin. Clin Cancer Res 1995;1:1595–601.

27. Vail DM, MacEwen EG, Kurzman ID, et al. Liposome-encapsulated muramyl tripeptide phosphatidylethanolamine adjuvant immunotherapy for splenic hemangiosarcoma in the dog: a randomized multi-institutional clinical trial. Clin Cancer Res 1995;1:1165–70.

28. Musser ML, Coto GM, Lingnan Y, et al. Pilot safety evaluation of doxorubicin chemotherapy combined with non-specific immunotherapy (Immunocidin®) for canine splenic hemangiosarcoma. PLoS One 2022;17:e0279594.

29. Arendt M, Nasir L, Morgan IM. Oncolytic gene therapy for canine cancers: teaching old dog viruses new tricks. Vet Comp Oncol 2009;7:153–61.

30. Smith BF, Curiel DT, Ternovoi VV, et al. Administration of a conditionally replicative oncolytic canine adenovirus in normal dogs. Cancer Biother Radiopharm 2006;21:601–6.

31. Le LP, Rivera AA, Glasgow JN, et al. Infectivity enhancement for adenoviral transduction of canine osteosarcoma cells. Gene Ther 2006;13:389–99.

32. Hemminki A, Kanerva A, Kremer EJ, et al. A canine conditionally replicating adenovirus for evaluating oncolytic virotherapy in a syngeneic animal model. Mol Ther 2003;7:163–73.

33. Suter SE, Chein MB, von M, et al. In vitro canine distemper virus infection of canine lymphoid cells: a prelude to oncolytic therapy for lymphoma. Clin Cancer Res 2005;11:1579–87.

34. Meyer T, Stockfleth E. Clinical investigations of Toll-like receptor agonists. Expet Opin Invest Drugs 2008;17:1051–65.

35. Gill VL, Bergman PJ, Baer KE, et al. Use of imiquimod 5% cream (Aldara™) in cats with multicentric squamous cell carcinoma in situ: 12 cases (2002-2005). Vet Comp Oncol 2008;6:55–64.

36. Peters-Kennedy J, Scott DW, Miller WH Jr. Apparent clinical resolution of pinnal actinic keratoses and squamous cell carcinoma in a cat using topical imiquimod 5% cream. J Feline Med Surg 2008;10(6):593–9.

37. Coyner K, Loeffler D. Topical imiquimod in the treatment of two cutaneous melanocytomas in a dog. Vet Dermatol 2012;23:145–149, e131.

38. Tateyama S, Priosoeryanto BP, Yamaguchi R, et al. In vitro growth inhibition activities of recombinant feline interferon on all lines derived from canine tumors. Res Vet Sci 1995;59:275–7.

39. Kruth SA. Biological response modifiers: Interferons, interleukins, recombinant products, liposomal products. Vet Clin North Am Small Anim Pract 1998;28: 269–95.

40. Whitley EM, Church Bird A, Zucker KE, et al. Modulation by canine interferon-gamma of major histocompatibility complex and tumor-associated antigen expression in canine mammary tumor and melanoma cell lines. Anticancer Res 1995;15:923–30.

41. Hampel V, Schwarz B, Kempf C, et al. Adjuvant immunotherapy of feline fibrosarcoma with recombinant feline interferon-omega. J Vet Intern Med 2007;21:1340–6.

42. Finocchiaro LM, Glikin GC. Cytokine-enhanced vaccine and suicide gene therapy as surgery adjuvant treatments for spontaneous canine melanoma. Gene Ther 2008;15:267–76.

43. Cutrera J, Torrero M, Shiomitsu K, et al. Intratumoral bleomycin and IL-12 electrochemogenetherapy for treating head and neck tumors in dogs. Methods Mol Biol 2008;423:319–25.

44. Finocchiaro LM, Fiszman GL, Karara AL, et al. Suicide gene and cytokines combined nonviral gene therapy for spontaneous canine melanoma. Cancer Gene Ther 2008;15:165–72.

45. Akhtar N, Padilla ML, Dickerson EB, et al. Interleukin-12 inhibits tumor growth in a novel angiogenesis canine hemangiosarcoma xenograft model. Neoplasia 2004;6:106–16.

46. Dickerson EB, Fosmire S, Padilla ML, et al. Potential to target dysregulated interleukin-2 receptor expression in canine lymphoid and hematopoietic malignancies as a model for human cancer. J Immunother 2002;25:36–45.

47. Okano F, Yamada K. Canine interleukin-18 induces apoptosis and enhances Fas ligand mRNA expression in a canine carcinoma cell line. Anticancer Res 2000; 20:3411–5.

48. Jahnke A, Hirschberger J, Fischer C, et al. Intra-tumoral gene delivery of feIL-2, feIFN-gamma and feGM-CSF using magnetofection as a neoadjuvant treatment option for feline fibrosarcomas: a phase-I study. J Vet Med A Physiol Pathol Clin Med 2007;54:599–606.

49. Dickerson EB, Akhtar N, Steinberg H, et al. Enhancement of the antiangiogenic activity of interleukin-12 by peptide targeted delivery of the cytokine to alphav-beta3 integrin. Mol Cancer Res 2004;2:663–73.

50. Finocchiaro LM, Fondello C, Gil-Cardeza ML, et al. Cytokine-Enhanced Vaccine and Interferon-beta plus Suicide Gene Therapy as Surgery Adjuvant Treatments for Spontaneous Canine Melanoma. Hum Gene Ther 2015;26:367–76.

51. Finocchiaro LME, Spector AIM, Agnetti L, et al. Combination of Suicide and Cytokine Gene Therapies as Surgery Adjuvant for Canine Mammary Carcinoma. Vet Sci 2018;5.

52. Tellado M, De Robertis M, Montagna D, et al. Electrochemotherapy Plus IL-2+IL-12 Gene Electrotransfer in Spontaneous Inoperable Stage III-IV Canine Oral Malignant Melanoma. Vaccines (Basel) 2023;11.

53. Brloznik M, Kranjc Brezar S, Boc N, et al. Results of Dynamic Contrast-Enhanced Ultrasound Correlate With Treatment Outcome in Canine Neoplasia Treated With Electrochemotherapy and Interleukin-12 Plasmid Electrotransfer. Front Vet Sci 2021;8:679073.

54. Dow S, Elmslie R, Kurzman I, et al. Phase I study of liposome-DNA complexes encoding the interleukin-2 gene in dogs with osteosarcoma lung metastases. Hum Gene Ther 2005;16:937–46.

55. Skubitz KM, Anderson PM. Inhalational interleukin-2 liposomes for pulmonary metastases: a phase I clinical trial. Anti Cancer Drugs 2000;11:555–63.

56. Khanna C, Hasz DE, Klausner JS, et al. Aerosol delivery of interleukin 2 liposomes is nontoxic and biologically effective: canine studies. Clin Cancer Res 1996;2:721–34.

57. Khanna C, Anderson PM, Hasz DE, et al. Interleukin-2 liposome inhalation therapy is safe and effective for dogs with spontaneous pulmonary metastases. Cancer 1997;79:1409–21.

58. Siddiqui F, Li CY, Zhang X, et al. Characterization of a recombinant adenovirus vector encoding heat-inducible feline interleukin-12 for use in hyperthermia-induced gene-therapy. Int J Hyperther 2006;22:117–34.

59. Jourdier TM, Moste C, Bonnet MC, et al. Local immunotherapy of spontaneous feline fibrosarcomas using recombinant poxviruses expressing interleukin 2 (IL2). Gene Ther 2003;10:2126–32.

60. Quintin-Colonna F, Devauchelle P, Fradelizi D, et al. Gene therapy of spontaneous canine melanoma and feline fibrosarcoma by intratumoral administration of histoincompatible cells expressing human interleukin-2. Gene Ther 1996;3: 1104–12.

61. Kamstock D, Guth A, Elmslie R, et al. Liposome-DNA complexes infused intravenously inhibit tumor angiogenesis and elicit antitumor activity in dogs with soft tissue sarcoma. Cancer Gene Ther 2006;13:306–17.

62. Junco JA, Basalto R, Fuentes F, et al. Gonadotrophin releasing hormone-based vaccine, an effective candidate for prostate cancer and other hormone-sensitive neoplasms. Adv Exp Med Biol 2008;617:581–7.

63. Chou PC, Chuang TF, Jan TR, et al. Effects of immunotherapy of IL-6 and IL-15 plasmids on transmissible venereal tumor in beagles. Vet Immunol Immunopathol 2009;130:25–34.

64. Chuang TF, Lee SC, Liao KW, et al. Electroporation-mediated IL-12 gene therapy in a transplantable canine cancer model. Int J Cancer 2009;125:698–707.

65. Finocchiaro LM, Glikin GC. Cytokine-enhanced vaccine and suicide gene therapy as surgery adjuvant treatments for spontaneous canine melanoma: 9 years of follow-up. Cancer Gene Ther 2012;19:852–61.

66. Takeuchi H, Konnai S, Maekawa N, et al. Canine Transforming Growth Factor-β Receptor 2-Ig: A Potential Candidate Biologic for Melanoma Treatment That Reverses Transforming Growth Factor-β1 Immunosuppression. Front Vet Sci 2021; 8:656715.

67. Seymour L, Bogaerts J, Perrone A, et al. iRECIST: guidelines for response criteria for use in trials testing immunotherapeutics. Lancet Oncol 2017;18:e143–52.

68. Bergman PJ. Anticancer vaccines. Vet Clin North Am Small Anim Pract 2007;37: 1111–9.

69. Beatty PL, Finn OJ. Preventing cancer by targeting abnormally expressed self-antigens: MUC1 vaccines for prevention of epithelial adenocarcinomas. Ann N Y Acad Sci 2013;1284:52–6.

70. Regan D, Guth A, Coy J, et al. Cancer immunotherapy in veterinary medicine: Current options and new developments. Vet J 2016;207:20–8.

71. Srisawat W, Nambooppha B, Pringproa K, et al. A Preliminary Study of the Cross-Reactivity of Canine MAGE-A with Hominid Monoclonal Antibody 6C1 in

Canine Mammary Gland Tumors: An Attractive Target for Cancer Diagnostic, Prognostic and Immunotherapeutic Development in Dogs. Vet Sci 2020;7.

72. Hogge GS, Burkholder JK, Culp J, et al. Preclinical development of human granulocyte-macrophage colony-stimulating factor-transfected melanoma cell vaccine using established canine cell lines and normal dogs. Cancer Gene Ther 1999;6:26–36.

73. Turek MM, Thamm DH, Mitzey A, et al. Human granulocyte & macrophage colony-stimulating factor DNA cationic-lipid complexed autologous tumour cell vaccination in the treatment of canine B-cell multicentric lymphoma. Vet Comp Oncol 2007;5:219–31.

74. Alexander AN, Huelsmeyer MK, Mitzey A, et al. Development of an allogeneic whole-cell tumor vaccine expressing xenogeneic gp100 and its implementation in a phase II clinical trial in canine patients with malignant melanoma. Cancer Immunol Immunother 2006;55:433–42.

75. U'Ren LW, Biller BJ, Elmslie RE, et al. Evaluation of a novel tumor vaccine in dogs with hemangiosarcoma. J Vet Intern Med 2007;21:113–20.

76. Bird RC, Deinnocentes P, Lenz S, et al. An allogeneic hybrid-cell fusion vaccine against canine mammary cancer. Vet Immunol Immunopathol 2008;123:289–304.

77. Kuntsi-Vaattovaara H, Verstraete FJM, Newsome JT, et al. Resolution of persistent oral papillomatosis in a dog after treatment with a recombinant canine oral papillomavirus vaccine. Vet Comp Oncol 2003;1:57–63.

78. Milner RJ, Salute M, Crawford C, et al. The immune response to disialoganglioside GD3 vaccination in normal dogs: a melanoma surface antigen vaccine. Vet Immunol Immunopathol 2006;114:273–84.

79. Marconato L, Frayssinet P, Rouquet N, et al. Randomized, placebo-controlled, double-blinded chemoimmunotherapy clinical trial in a pet dog model of diffuse large B-cell lymphoma. Clin Cancer Res 2014;20:668–77.

80. Suckow MA. Cancer vaccines: harnessing the potential of anti-tumor immunity. Vet J 2013;198:28–33.

81. Epple LM, Bemis LT, Cavanaugh RP, et al. Prolonged remission of advanced bronchoalveolar adenocarcinoma in a dog treated with autologous, tumour-derived chaperone-rich cell lysate (CRCL) vaccine. Int J Hyperther 2013;29:390–8.

82. Andersen BM, Pluhar GE, Seiler CE, et al. Vaccination for invasive canine meningioma induces in situ production of antibodies capable of antibody-dependent cell-mediated cytotoxicity. Cancer Res 2013;73:2987–97.

83. Yannelli JR, Wouda R, Masterson TJ, et al. Development of an autologous canine cancer vaccine system for resectable malignant tumors in dogs. Vet Immunol Immunopathol 2016;182:95–100.

84. Marconato L, Stefanello D, Sabattini S, et al. Enhanced therapeutic effect of APAVAC immunotherapy in combination with dose-intense chemotherapy in dogs with advanced indolent B-cell lymphoma. Vaccine 2015;33:5080–6.

85. Weir C, Hudson AL, Moon E, et al. Streptavidin: a novel immunostimulant for the selection and delivery of autologous and syngeneic tumor vaccines. Cancer Immunol Res 2014;2:469–79.

86. Weir C, Oksa A, Millar J, et al. The Safety of an Adjuvanted Autologous Cancer Vaccine Platform in Canine Cancer Patients. Vet Sci 2018;5.

87. Garcia JS, Nowosh V, LÃ³pez RVM, et al. Association of Systemic Inflammatory and Immune Indices With Survival in Canine Patients With Oral Melanoma, Treated With Experimental Immunotherapy Alone or Experimental Immunotherapy Plus Metronomic Chemotherapy. Front Vet Sci 2022;9:888411.

88. Magee K, Marsh IR, Turek MM, et al. Safety and feasibility of an in situ vaccination and immunomodulatory targeted radionuclide combination immunoradiotherapy approach in a comparative (companion dog) setting. PLoS One 2021;16:e0255798.

89. Riccardo F, Tarone L, Camerino M, et al. Antigen mimicry as an effective strategy to induce CSPG4-targeted immunity in dogs with oral melanoma: a veterinary trial. J Immunother Cancer 2022;10.

90. Kamstock D, Elmslie R, Thamm D, et al. Evaluation of a xenogeneic VEGF vaccine in dogs with soft tissue sarcoma. Cancer Immunol Immunother 2007;56:1299–309.

91. Yu WY, Chuang TF, Guichard C, et al. Chicken HSP70 DNA vaccine inhibits tumor growth in a canine cancer model. Vaccine 2011;29:3489–500.

92. Impellizeri JA, Ciliberto G, Aurisicchio L. Electro-gene-transfer as a new tool for cancer immunotherapy in animals. Vet Comp Oncol 2014;12:310–8.

93. Denies S, Cicchelero L, Polis I, et al. Immunogenicity and safety of xenogeneic vascular endothelial growth factor receptor-2 DNA vaccination in mice and dogs. Oncotarget 2016;7:10905–16.

94. Gabai V, Venanzi FM, Bagashova E, et al. Pilot study of p62 DNA vaccine in dogs with mammary tumors. Oncotarget 2014;5:12803–10.

95. Riccardo F, Iussich S, Maniscalco L, et al. CSPG4-specific immunity and survival prolongation in dogs with oral malignant melanoma immunized with human CSPG4 DNA. Clin Cancer Res 2014;20:3753–62.

96. Gibson HM, Veenstra JJ, Jones R, et al. Induction of HER2 Immunity in Outbred Domestic Cats by DNA Electrovaccination. Cancer Immunol Res 2015;3:777–86.

97. Piras LA, Riccardo F, Iussich S, et al. Prolongation of survival of dogs with oral malignant melanoma treated by en bloc surgical resection and adjuvant CSPG4-antigen electrovaccination. Vet Comp Oncol 2017;15:996–1013.

98. Engbersen DJM, van Beijnum JR, Roos A, et al. Vaccination against Extracellular Vimentin for Treatment of Urothelial Cancer of the Bladder in Client-Owned Dogs. Cancers 2023;15.

99. Tarone L, Giacobino D, Camerino M, et al. A chimeric human/dog-DNA vaccine against CSPG4 induces immunity with therapeutic potential in comparative preclinical models of osteosarcoma. Mol Ther 2023;31:2342–59.

100. Ammons DT, Guth A, Rozental AJ, et al. Reprogramming the Canine Glioma Microenvironment with Tumor Vaccination plus Oral Losartan and Propranolol Induces Objective Responses. Cancer Res Commun 2022;2:1657–67.

101. Camerino M, Giacobino D, Manassero L, et al. Prognostic impact of bone invasion in canine oral malignant melanoma treated by surgery and anti-CSPG4 vaccination: A retrospective study on 68 cases (2010-2020). Vet Comp Oncol 2022;20:189–97.

102. Giacobino D, Camerino M, Riccardo F, et al. Difference in outcome between curative intent vs marginal excision as a first treatment in dogs with oral malignant melanoma and the impact of adjuvant CSPG4-DNA electrovaccination: A retrospective study on 155 cases. Vet Comp Oncol 2021;19:651–60.

103. Doyle HA, Koski RA, Bonafé N, et al. Epidermal growth factor receptor peptide vaccination induces cross-reactive immunity to human EGFR, HER2, and HER3. Cancer Immunol Immunother 2018;67:1559–69.

104. Doyle HA, Gee RJ, Masters TD, et al. Vaccine-induced ErbB (EGFR/HER2)-specific immunity in spontaneous canine cancer. Transl Oncol 2021;14:101205.

105. von EH, Sadeghi A, Carlsson B, et al. Efficient adenovector CD40 ligand immunotherapy of canine malignant melanoma. J Immunother 2008;31:377–84.

106. Johnston KB, Monteiro JM, Schultz LD, et al. Protection of beagle dogs from mucosal challenge with canine oral papillomavirus by immunization with recombinant adenoviruses expressing codon-optimized early genes. Virology 2005; 336:208–18.

107. Thacker EE, Nakayama M, Smith BF, et al. A genetically engineered adenovirus vector targeted to CD40 mediates transduction of canine dendritic cells and promotes antigen-specific immune responses in vivo. Vaccine 2009;27:7116–24.

108. Peruzzi D, Mesiti G, Ciliberto G, et al. Telomerase and HER-2/neu as targets of genetic cancer vaccines in dogs. Vaccine 2010;28:1201–8.

109. Gavazza A, Lubas G, Fridman A, et al. Safety and efficacy of a genetic vaccine targeting telomerase plus chemotherapy for the therapy of canine B-cell lymphoma. Hum Gene Ther 2013;24:728–38.

110. Autio KP, Ruotsalainen JJ, Anttila MO, et al. Attenuated Semliki Forest virus for cancer treatment in dogs: safety assessment in two laboratory Beagles. BMC Vet Res 2015;11:170.

111. Impellizeri JA, Gavazza A, Greissworth E, et al. Tel-eVax: a genetic vaccine targeting telomerase for treatment of canine lymphoma. J Transl Med 2018;16:349.

112. Hoopes PJ, Wagner RJ, Duval K, et al. Treatment of Canine Oral Melanoma with Nanotechnology-Based Immunotherapy and Radiation. Mol Pharm 2018;15: 3717–22.

113. Sanchez D, Cesarman-Maus G, Amador-Molina A, et al. Oncolytic viruses for canine cancer treatment. Cancers 2018;10.

114. Cejalvo T, Perise-Barrios AJ, Del P I, et al. Remission of Spontaneous Canine Tumors after Systemic Cellular Viroimmunotherapy. Cancer Res 2018;78:4891–901.

115. Hoopes PJ, Moodie KL, Petryk AA, et al. Hypo-fractionated Radiation, Magnetic Nanoparticle Hyperthermia and a Viral Immunotherapy Treatment of Spontaneous Canine Cancer. Proc SPIE-Int Soc Opt Eng 2017;10066.

116. Makielski KM, Sarver AL, Henson MS, et al. Oncolytic vesicular stomatitis virus is safe and provides a survival benefit for dogs with naturally occurring osteosarcoma. bioRxiv 2023;31:100736.

117. Martín-Carrasco C, Delgado-Bonet P, Tomeo-Martín BD, et al. Safety and Efficacy of an Oncolytic Adenovirus as an Immunotherapy for Canine Cancer Patients. Vet Sci 2022;9.

118. Alonso-Miguel D, Valdivia G, Guerrera D, et al. Neoadjuvant in situ vaccination with cowpea mosaic virus as a novel therapy against canine inflammatory mammary cancer. J Immunother Cancer 2022;10.

119. Saellstrom S, Sadeghi A, Eriksson E, et al. Adenoviral CD40 Ligand Immunotherapy in 32 Canine Malignant Melanomas-Long-Term Follow Up. Front Vet Sci 2021;8:695222.

120. Gyorffy S, Rodriguez-Lecompte JC, Woods JP, et al. Bone marrow-derived dendritic cell vaccination of dogs with naturally occurring melanoma by using human gp100 antigen. J Vet Intern Med 2005;19:56–63.

121. Tamura K, Arai H, Ueno E, et al. Comparison of dendritic cell-mediated immune responses among canine malignant cells. J Vet Med Sci 2007;69:925–30.

122. Tamura K, Yamada M, Isotani M, et al. Induction of dendritic cell-mediated immune responses against canine malignant melanoma cells. Vet J 2008;175: 126–9.

123. Rodriguez-Lecompte JC, Kruth S, Gyorffy S, et al. Cell-based cancer gene therapy: breaking tolerance or inducing autoimmunity? Anim Health Res Rev 2004; 5:227–34.

124. Kyte JA, Mu L, Aamdal S, et al. Phase I/II trial of melanoma therapy with dendritic cells transfected with autologous tumor-mRNA. Cancer Gene Ther 2006; 13:905–18.

125. Mason NJ, Coughlin CM, Overley B, et al. RNA-loaded CD40-activated B cells stimulate antigen-specific T-cell responses in dogs with spontaneous lymphoma. Gene Ther 2008;15:955–65.

126. Sorenmo KU, Krick E, Coughlin CM, et al. CD40-activated B cell cancer vaccine improves second clinical remission and survival in privately owned dogs with non-Hodgkin's lymphoma. PLoS One 2011;6:e24167.

127. Bird RC, Deinnocentes P, Church Bird AE, et al. An autologous dendritic cell canine mammary tumor hybrid-cell fusion vaccine. Cancer Immunol Immunother 2011;60:87–97.

128. Bird RC, DeInnocentes P, Church Bird AE, et al. Autologous hybrid cell fusion vaccine in a spontaneous intermediate model of breast carcinoma. J Vet Sci 2019;20:e48.

129. Hernandez-Granados AJ, Franco-Molina MA, Coronado-Cerda EE, et al. Immunogenic potential of three transmissible venereal tumor cell lysates to prime canine-dendritic cells for cancer immunotherapy. Res Vet Sci 2018;121:23–30.

130. O'Connor CM, Sheppard S, Hartline CA, et al. Adoptive T-cell therapy improves treatment of canine non-Hodgkin lymphoma post chemotherapy. Sci Rep 2012; 2:249.

131. Gareau A, Ripoll AZ, Suter SE. A Retrospective Analysis: Autologous Peripheral Blood Hematopoietic Stem Cell Transplant Combined With Adoptive T-Cell Therapy for the Treatment of High-Grade B-Cell Lymphoma in Ten Dogs. Front Vet Sci 2021;8:787373.

132. Kisseberth WC, Lee DA. Adoptive Natural Killer Cell Immunotherapy for Canine Osteosarcoma. Front Vet Sci 2021;8:672361.

133. Lucroy MD, Clauson RM, Suckow MA, et al. Evaluation of an autologous cancer vaccine for the treatment of metastatic canine hemangiosarcoma: a preliminary study. BMC Vet Res 2020;16:447.

134. Lucroy MD, Kugler AM, El-Tayyeb F, et al. Field safety experience with an autologous cancer vaccine in tumor-bearing cats: a retrospective study of 117 cases (2015-2020). J Feline Med Surg 2022;24:493–9.

135. Goodrich RP, Weston J, Hartson L, et al. Pilot Acute Safety Evaluation of Innocell™ Cancer Immunotherapy in Canine Subjects. J Immunol Res 2020;2020:7142375.

136. Sharma P, Wagner K, Wolchok JD, et al. Novel cancer immunotherapy agents with survival benefit: recent successes and next steps. Nat Rev Cancer 2011; 11:805–12.

137. Singh S, Kumar N, Dwiwedi P, et al. Monoclonal Antibodies: A Review, Curr Clin Pharmacol 2018;13(2):85–99.

138. Proksch SF, Matthysen CP, Jardine JE, et al. Developing a translational murine-to-canine pathway for an IL-2/agonist anti-CD40 antibody cancer immunotherapy. Vet Comp Oncol 2022;20:602–12.

139. Gameiro A, Nascimento C, Correia J, et al. HER2-Targeted Immunotherapy and Combined Protocols Showed Promising Antiproliferative Effects in Feline Mammary Carcinoma Cell-Based Models. Cancers 2021;13.

140. Ladjemi MZ. Anti-idiotypic antibodies as cancer vaccines: achievements and future improvements. Front Oncol 2012;2:158.

141. Thomas A, Teicher BA, Hassan R. Antibody-drug conjugates for cancer therapy. Lancet Oncol 2016;17:e254–62.

142. Ross SL, Sherman M, McElroy PL, et al. Bispecific T cell engager (BiTE(R)) anti-body constructs can mediate bystander tumor cell killing. PLoS One 2017;12: e0183390.

143. Strohl WR. Current progress in innovative engineered antibodies. Protein Cell 2018;9(1):86–120.

144. Grillo-Lopez AJ, Hedrick E, Rashford M, et al. Rituximab: ongoing and future clinical development. Semin Oncol 2002;29:105–12.

145. Saxena A, Wu D. Advances in Therapeutic Fc Engineering - Modulation of IgG-Associated Effector Functions and Serum Half-life. Front Immunol 2016;7:580.

146. Weiskopf K, Anderson KL, Ito D, et al. Eradication of Canine Diffuse Large B-Cell Lymphoma in a Murine Xenograft Model with CD47 Blockade and Anti-CD20. Cancer Immunol Res 2016;4:1072–87.

147. Jain S, Aresu L, Comazzi S, et al. The Development of a Recombinant scFv Monoclonal Antibody Targeting Canine CD20 for Use in Comparative Medicine. PLoS One 2016;11:e0148366.

148. Ito D, Brewer S, Modiano JF, et al. Development of a novel anti-canine CD20 monoclonal antibody with diagnostic and therapeutic potential. Leuk Lymphoma 2015;56:219–25.

149. Rue SM, Eckelman BP, Efe JA, et al. Identification of a candidate therapeutic antibody for treatment of canine B-cell lymphoma. Vet Immunol Immunopathol 2015;164:148–59.

150. Kano R, Inoiue C, Okano H, et al. Canine CD20 gene. Vet Immunol Immunopathol 2005;108:265–8.

151. Jubala CM, Wojcieszyn JW, Valli VE, et al. CD20 expression in normal canine B cells and in canine non-Hodgkin lymphoma. Vet Pathol 2005;42:468–76.

152. Impellizeri JA, Howell K, McKeever KP, et al. The role of rituximab in the treatment of canine lymphoma: an ex vivo evaluation. Vet J 2006;171:556–8.

153. Dias JNR, Almeida A, André AS, et al. Characterization of the canine CD20 as a therapeutic target for comparative passive immunotherapy. Sci Rep 2022;12: 2678.

154. Sakai O, Ogino S, Tsukui T, et al. Development of a monoclonal antibody for the detection of anti-canine CD20 chimeric antigen receptor expression on canine CD20 chimeric antigen receptor-transduced T cells. J Vet Med Sci 2021;83: 1495–9.

155. Musser ML, Clifford CA, Bergman PJ, et al. Randomised trial evaluating chemotherapy alone or chemotherapy and a novel monoclonal antibody for canine T-cell lymphoma: A multicentre US study. Vet Rec Open 2022;9:e49.

156. London CA, Gardner HL, Rippy S, et al. KTN0158, a Humanized Anti-KIT Monoclonal Antibody, Demonstrates Biologic Activity against both Normal and Malignant Canine Mast Cells. Clin Cancer Res 2017;23:2565–74.

157. Adelfinger M, Bessler S, Frentzen A, et al. Preclinical Testing Oncolytic Vaccinia Virus Strain GLV-5b451 Expressing an Anti-VEGF Single-Chain Antibody for Canine Cancer Therapy. Viruses 2015;7:4075–92.

158. Wagner S, Maibaum D, Pich A, et al. Verification of a canine PSMA (FolH1) antibody. Anticancer Res 2015;35:145–8.

159. Singer J, Fazekas J, Wang W, et al. Generation of a canine anti-EGFR (ErbB-1) antibody for passive immunotherapy in dog cancer patients. Mol Cancer Therapeut 2014;13:1777–90.

160. Michishita M, Uto T, Nakazawa R, et al. Antitumor effect of bevacizumab in a xenograft model of canine hemangiopericytoma. J Pharmacol Sci 2013;121: 339–42.

161. Michishita M, Ohtsuka A, Nakahira R, et al. Anti-tumor effect of bevacizumab on a xenograft model of feline mammary carcinoma. J Vet Med Sci 2016;78:685–9.

162. Shahabi V, Seavey MM, Maciag PC, et al. Development of a live and highly attenuated Listeria monocytogenes-based vaccine for the treatment of Her2/neu-overexpressing cancers in human. Cancer Gene Ther 2011;18:53–62.

163. Fazekas J, Furdos I, Singer J, et al. Why man's best friend, the dog, could also benefit from an anti-HER-2 vaccine. Oncol Lett 2016;12:2271–6.

164. Mason NJ, Gnanandarajah JS, Engiles JB, et al. Immunotherapy with a HER2-Targeting Listeria Induces HER2-Specific Immunity and Demonstrates Potential Therapeutic Effects in a Phase I Trial in Canine Osteosarcoma. Clin Cancer Res 2016;22:4380–90.

165. Musser ML, Berger EP, Parsons C, et al. Vaccine strain Listeria monocytogenes abscess in a dog: a case report. BMC Vet Res 2019;15:467.

166. Musser ML, Berger EP, Tripp CD, et al. Safety evaluation of the canine osteosarcoma vaccine, live Listeria vector. Vet Comp Oncol 2021;19:92–8.

167. Bergman PJ, McKnight J, Novosad A, et al. Long-term survival of dogs with advanced malignant melanoma after DNA vaccination with xenogeneic human tyrosinase: a phase I trial. Clin Cancer Res 2003;9:1284–90.

168. Bergman PJ, Camps-Palau MA, McKnight JA, et al. Development of a xenogeneic DNA vaccine program for canine malignant melanoma at the Animal Medical Center. Vaccine 2006;24:4582–5.

169. Smedley RC, Lamoureux J, Sledge DG, et al. Immunohistochemical diagnosis of canine oral amelanotic melanocytic neoplasms. Vet Pathol 2011;48:32–40.

170. Phillips JC, Lembcke LM, Noltenius CE, et al. Evaluation of tyrosinase expression in canine and equine melanocytic tumors. Am J Vet Res 2012;73:272–8.

171. Cangul IT, van Garderen E, van der Poel HJ, et al. Tyrosinase gene expression in clear cell sarcoma indicates a melanocytic origin: insight from the first reported canine case. Apmis 1999;107:982–8.

172. Ramos-Vara JA, Beissenherz ME, Miller MA, et al. Retrospective study of 338 canine oral melanomas with clinical, histologic, and immunohistochemical review of 129 cases. Vet Pathol JID 2000;37:597–608.

173. Ramos-Vara JA, Miller MA. Immunohistochemical identification of canine melanocytic neoplasms with antibodies to melanocytic antigen PNL2 and tyrosinase: comparison with Melan A. Vet Pathol 2011;48:443–50.

174. de Vries TJ, Smeets M, de Graaf R, et al. Expression of gp100, MART-1, tyrosinase, and S100 in paraffin-embedded primary melanomas and locoregional, lymph node, and visceral metastases: implications for diagnosis and immunotherapy. A study conducted by the EORTC Melanoma Cooperative Group. J Pathol 2001;193:13–20.

175. Gradilone A, Gazzaniga P, Ribuffo D, et al. Prognostic significance of tyrosinase expression in sentinel lymph node biopsy for ultra-thin, thin, and thick melanomas. Eur Rev Med Pharmacol Sci 2012;16:1367–76.

176. Liao JC, Gregor P, Wolchok JD, et al. Vaccination with human tyrosinase DNA induces antibody responses in dogs with advanced melanoma. Cancer Immun 2006;6:8.

177. Goubier A, Fuhrmann L, Forest L, et al. Superiority of needle-free transdermal plasmid delivery for the induction of antigen-specific IFNgamma T cell responses in the dog. Vaccine 2008;26:2186–90.

178. Grosenbaugh DA, Leard AT, Bergman PJ, et al. Safety and efficacy of a xenogeneic DNA vaccine encoding for human tyrosinase as adjunctive treatment

for oral malignant melanoma in dogs following surgical excision of the primary tumor. Am J Vet Res 2011;72:1631–8.

179. Zuleger CL, Kang C, Ranheim EA, et al. Pilot study of safety and feasibility of DNA microseeding for treatment of spontaneous canine melanoma. Vet Med Sci 2017;3:134–45.

180. Herzog A, Buchholz J, Ruess-Melzer K, et al. [Combined use of irradiation and DNA tumor vaccine to treat canine oral malignant melanoma: a pilot study]. Schweiz Arch Tierheilkd 2013;155:135–42.

181. Ottnod JM, Smedley RC, Walshaw R, et al. A retrospective analysis of the efficacy of Oncept vaccine for the adjunct treatment of canine oral malignant melanoma. Vet Comp Oncol 2013;11:219–29.

182. Verganti S, Berlato D, Blackwood L, et al. Use of Oncept melanoma vaccine in 69 canine oral malignant melanomas in the UK. J Small Anim Pract 2017; 58:10–6.

183. Treggiari E, Grant JP, North SM. A retrospective review of outcome and survival following surgery and adjuvant xenogeneic DNA vaccination in 32 dogs with oral malignant melanoma. J Vet Med Sci 2016;78:845–50.

184. McLean JL, Lobetti RG. Use of the melanoma vaccine in 38 dogs: The South African experience. J S Afr Vet Assoc 2015;86:1246.

185. Boston SE, Lu X, Culp WT, et al. Efficacy of systemic adjuvant therapies administered to dogs after excision of oral malignant melanomas: 151 cases (2001-2012). J Am Vet Med Assoc 2014;245:401–7.

186. Wolchok JD, Yuan J, Houghton AN, et al. Safety and immunogenicity of tyrosinase DNA vaccines in patients with melanoma. Mol Ther 2007;15:2044–50.

187. Perales MA, Yuan J, Powel S, et al. Phase I/II study of GM-CSF DNA as an adjuvant for a multipeptide cancer vaccine in patients with advanced melanoma. Mol Ther 2008;16:2022–9.

188. Yuan J, Ku GY, Gallardo HF, et al. Safety and immunogenicity of a human and mouse gp100 DNA vaccine in a phase I trial of patients with melanoma. Cancer Immun 2009;9:5.

189. Ginsberg BA, Gallardo HF, Rasalan TS, et al. Immunologic response to xenogeneic gp100 DNA in melanoma patients: comparison of particle-mediated epidermal delivery with intramuscular injection. Clin Cancer Res 2010;16:4057–65.

190. Manley CA, Leibman NF, Wolchok JD, et al. Xenogeneic Murine Tyrosinase DNA Vaccine for Malignant Melanoma of the Digit of Dogs. J Vet Intern Med 2011; 25(1):94–9.

191. Phillips JCBJ, Lembcke LM, Grosenbaugh DA, et al. Evaluation of Needle-Free Injection Devices for Intramuscular Vaccination in Horses. J Eq VetSci 2011;31: 738–43.

192. Sarbu L, Kitchell BE, Bergman PJ. Safety of administering the canine melanoma DNA vaccine (Oncept) to cats with malignant melanoma - a retrospective study. J Feline Med Surg 2017;19(2):224–30.

193. Mangold BJ, Flower JE, Burgess KE, et al. Use of a canine melanoma vaccine in the management of malignant melanoma in an African penguin (Spheniscus demersus). J Am Vet Med Assoc 2021;260:455–60.

194. Chu PY, Pan SL, Liu CH, et al. KIT gene exon 11 mutations in canine malignant melanoma. Vet J 2013;196:226–30.

195. Murakami A, Mori T, Sakai H, et al. Analysis of KIT expression and KIT exon 11 mutations in canine oral malignant melanomas. Vet Comp Oncol 2011;9:219–24.

196. Gillard M, Cadieu E, De BC, et al. Naturally occurring melanomas in dogs as models for non-UV pathways of human melanomas. Pigment Cell Melanoma Res 2014;27:90–102.

197. Demaria S, Formenti SC. The abscopal effect 67 years later: from a side story to center stage. Br J Radiol 2020;93:20200042.

198. Peggs KS, Quezada SA, Korman AJ, et al. Principles and use of anti-CTLA4 antibody in human cancer immunotherapy. Curr Opin Immunol 2006;18:206–13.

199. Graves SS, Stone D, Loretz C, et al. Establishment of long-term tolerance to SRBC in dogs by recombinant canine CTLA4-Ig. Transplantation 2009;88:317–22.

200. Callahan MK, Wolchok JD. At the bedside: CTLA-4- and PD-1-blocking antibodies in cancer immunotherapy. J Leukoc Biol 2013;94:41–53.

201. Biller BJ, Elmslie RE, Burnett RC, et al. Use of FoxP3 expression to identify regulatory T cells in healthy dogs and dogs with cancer. Vet Immunol Immunopathol 2007;116:69–78.

202. O'Neill K, Guth A, Biller B, et al. Changes in regulatory T cells in dogs with cancer and associations with tumor type. J Vet Intern Med 2009;23:875–81.

203. Sherger M, Kisseberth W, London C, et al. Identification of myeloid derived suppressor cells in the peripheral blood of tumor bearing dogs. BMC Vet Res 2012; 8:209.

204. Maeda S, Motegi T, Iio A, et al. Anti-CCR4 treatment depletes regulatory T cells and leads to clinical activity in a canine model of advanced prostate cancer. J Immunother Cancer 2022;10.

205. Thamm DH. Interactions between radiation therapy and immunotherapy: the best of two worlds? Vet Comp Oncol 2006;4:189–97.

206. Walter CU, Biller BJ, Lana SE, et al. Effects of chemotherapy on immune responses in dogs with cancer. J Vet Intern Med 2006;20:342–7.

207. Emens LA, Jaffee EM. Leveraging the activity of tumor vaccines with cytotoxic chemotherapy. Cancer Res 2005;65:8059–64.

208. Emens LA, Asquith JM, Leatherman JM, et al. Timed sequential treatment with cyclophosphamide, doxorubicin, and an allogeneic granulocyte-macrophage colony-stimulating factor-secreting breast tumor vaccine: a chemotherapy dose-ranging factorial study of safety and immune activation. J Clin Oncol 2009;27: 5911–8.

209. Pfannenstiel LW, Lam SS, Emens LA, et al. Paclitaxel enhances early dendritic cell maturation and function through TLR4 signaling in mice. Cell Immunol 2010;263:79–87.

210. Callahan MK, Wolchok JD, Allison JP. Anti-CTLA-4 antibody therapy: immune monitoring during clinical development of a novel immunotherapy. Semin Oncol 2010;37:473–84.

211. Ott PA, Hodi FS, Kaufman HL, et al. Combination immunotherapy: a road map. J Immunother Cancer 2017;5:16.

212. Hellmann MD, Friedman CF, Wolchok JD. Combinatorial Cancer Immunotherapies. Adv Immunol 2016;130:251–77.

213. Le D, Uram J, Wang H, et al. PD-1 Blockade in Tumors with Mismatch-Repair Deficiency. N Engl J Med 2015;372:2509–20.

214. Karaki S, Anson M, Tran T, et al. Is there still room for cancer vaccines at the era of checkpoint inhibitors, 4. Basel: Vaccines; 2016.

215. Lai X, Friedman A. Combination therapy of cancer with cancer vaccine and immune checkpoint inhibitors: A mathematical model. PLoS One 2017;12: e0178479.

216. Pinto C, Aluai-Cunha C, Santos A. The human and animals' malignant melanoma: comparative tumor models and the role of microbiome in dogs and humans. Melanoma Res 2023;33:87–103.

217. Yuasa T, Masuda H, Yamamoto S, et al. Biomarkers to predict prognosis and response to checkpoint inhibitors. Int J Clin Oncol 2017;22:629–34.

218. Khagi Y, Kurzrock R, Patel SP. Next generation predictive biomarkers for immune checkpoint inhibition. Cancer Metastasis Rev 2017;36:179–90.

219. Ott PA, Hu Z, Keskin DB, et al. An immunogenic personal neoantigen vaccine for patients with melanoma. Nature 2017;547:217–21.

220. Yang JC, Rosenberg SA. Adoptive T-Cell Therapy for Cancer. Adv Immunol 2016;130:279–94.

221. Jackson HJ, Rafiq S, Brentjens RJ. Driving CAR T-cells forward. Nat Rev Clin Oncol 2016;13:370–83.

222. Yun K, Siegler EL, Kenderian SS. Who wins the combat, CAR or TCR? Leukemia 2023;37(10):1953–62.

223. Cutmore LC, Marshall JF. Current perspectives on the use of off the shelf CAR-T/ NK cells for the treatment of cancer. Cancers 2021;13.

224. Flesner BK, Wood GW, Gayheart-Walsten P, et al. Autologous cancer cell vaccination, adoptive T-cell transfer, and interleukin-2 administration results in long-term survival for companion dogs with osteosarcoma. J Vet Intern Med 2020; 34:2056–67.

225. Bergman PJ, MacEwen EG, Kurzman ID, et al. Amputation and carboplatin for treatment of dogs with osteosarcoma: 48 cases (1991 to 1993). J Vet Intern Med 1996;10:76–81.

226. Skorupski KA, Uhl JM, Szivek A, et al. Carboplatin versus alternating carboplatin and doxorubicin for the adjuvant treatment of canine appendicular osteosarcoma: a randomized, phase III trial. Vet Comp Oncol 2016;14(1):81–7.

227. Selmic LE, Burton JH, Thamm DH, et al. Comparison of Carboplatin and Doxorubicin-based chemotherapy protocols in 470 dogs after amputation for treatment of appendicular osteosarcoma. J Vet Intern Med 2014;28:554–63.

228. LeBlanc AK, Mazcko CN, Cherukuri A, et al. Adjuvant Sirolimus Does Not Improve Outcome in Pet Dogs Receiving Standard-of-Care Therapy for Appendicular Osteosarcoma: A Prospective, Randomized Trial of 324 Dogs. Clin Cancer Res 2021;27:3005–16.

229. Phillips B, Powers BE, Dernell WS, et al. Use of single-agent carboplatin as adjuvant or neoadjuvant therapy in conjunction with amputation for appendicular osteosarcoma in dogs. J Am Anim Hosp Assoc 2009;45:33–8.

230. Coy J, Caldwell A, Chow L, et al. PD-1 expression by canine T cells and functional effects of PD-1 blockade. Vet Comp Oncol 2017;15(4):1487–502.

231. Maekawa N, Konnai S, Okagawa T, et al. Immunohistochemical Analysis of PD-L1 Expression in Canine Malignant Cancers and PD-1 Expression on Lymphocytes in Canine Oral Melanoma. PLoS One 2016;11:e0157176.

232. Maekawa N, Konnai S, Takagi S, et al. A canine chimeric monoclonal antibody targeting PD-L1 and its clinical efficacy in canine oral malignant melanoma or undifferentiated sarcoma. Sci Rep 2017;7:8951.

233. Shosu K, Sakurai M, Inoue K, et al. Programmed Cell Death Ligand 1 Expression in Canine Cancer. In Vivo 2016;30:195–204.

234. Chiku VM, Silva KL, de Almeida BF, et al. PD-1 function in apoptosis of T lymphocytes in canine visceral leishmaniasis. Immunobiology 2016;221:879–88.

235. Tagawa M, Maekawa N, Konnai S, et al. Evaluation of Costimulatory Molecules in Peripheral Blood Lymphocytes of Canine Patients with Histiocytic Sarcoma. PLoS One 2016;11:e0150030.

236. Esch KJ, Juelsgaard R, Martinez PA, et al. Programmed death 1-mediated T cell exhaustion during visceral leishmaniasis impairs phagocyte function. J Immunol 2013;191:5542–50.

237. Folkl A, Wen X, Kuczynski E, et al. Feline programmed death and its ligand: characterization and changes with feline immunodeficiency virus infection. Vet Immunol Immunopathol 2010;134:107–14.

238. Kumar SR, Kim DY, Henry CJ, et al. Programmed death ligand 1 is expressed in canine B cell lymphoma and downregulated by MEK inhibitors. Vet Comp Oncol 2017;15(4):1527–36.

239. Smith JB, Panjwani MK, Schutsky K, et al. Feasibility and safety of cCD20 RNA CAR-bearing T cell therapy for the treatment of canine B cell malignancies. J Immunother Cancer 2015;3:123.

240. Panjwani MK, Smith JB, Schutsky K, et al. Feasibility and Safety of RNA-transfected CD20-specific Chimeric Antigen Receptor T Cells in Dogs with Spontaneous B Cell Lymphoma. Mol Ther 2016;24:1602–14.

241. Anderson KL, Modiano JF. Progress in Adaptive Immunotherapy for Cancer in Companion Animals: Success on the Path to a Cure. Vet Sci 2015;2:363–87.

242. Mata M, Vera J, Gerken C, et al. Towards immunotherapy with redirected T cells in a large animal model: Ex vivo activation, expansion, and genetic modification of canine T cells. J Immunother 2014;37:407–15.

243. Mie K, Shimada T, Akiyoshi H, et al. Change in peripheral blood lymphocyte count in dogs following adoptive immunotherapy using lymphokine-activated T killer cells combined with palliative tumor resection. Vet Immunol Immunopathol 2016;177:58–63.

244. Kurupati RK, Zhou X, Xiang Z, et al. Safety and immunogenicity of a potential checkpoint blockade vaccine for canine melanoma. Cancer Immunol Immunother 2018;67:1533–44.

245. Nemoto Y, Shosu K, Okuda M, et al. Development and characterization of monoclonal antibodies against canine PD-1 and PD-L1. Vet Immunol Immunopathol 2018;198:19–25.

246. Canter RJ, Grossenbacher SK, Foltz JA, et al. Radiotherapy enhances natural killer cell cytotoxicity and localization in pre-clinical canine sarcomas and first-in-dog clinical trial. J Immunother Cancer 2017;5:98.

247. Sirivisoot S, Boonkrai C, Wongtangprasert T, et al. Development and characterization of mouse anti-canine PD-L1 monoclonal antibodies and their expression in canine tumors by immunohistochemistry in vitro. Vet Q 2023;43:1–9.

248. Oh W, Kim AMJ, Dhawan D, et al. Development of an Anti-canine PD-L1 Antibody and Caninized PD-L1 Mouse Model as Translational Research Tools for the Study of Immunotherapy in Humans. Cancer Res Commun 2023;3:860–73.

249. Talavera Guillén NC, Barboza de Nardi A, Noleto de Paiva F, et al. Clinical Implications of Immune Checkpoints and the RANK/RANK-L Signaling Pathway in High-Grade Canine Mast Cell Tumors. Animals (Basel) 2023;13.

250. Deguchi T, Maekawa N, Konnai S, et al. Enhanced Systemic Antitumour Immunity by Hypofractionated Radiotherapy and Anti-PD-L1 Therapy in Dogs with Pulmonary Metastatic Oral Malignant Melanoma. Cancers 2023;15.

251. Xu S, Xie J, Wang S, et al. Reversing stage III oral adenocarcinoma in a dog treated with anti-canine PD-1 therapeutic antibody: a case report. Front Vet Sci 2023;10:1144869.

252. Forsberg EMV, Riise R, Saellström S, et al. Treatment with Anti-HER2 Chimeric Antigen Receptor Tumor-Infiltrating Lymphocytes (CAR-TILs) Is Safe and Associated with Antitumor Efficacy in Mice and Companion Dogs. Cancers 2023;15.

253. Stevenson VB, Klahn S, LeRoith T, et al. Canine melanoma: A review of diagnostics and comparative mechanisms of disease and immunotolerance in the era of the immunotherapies. Front Vet Sci 2022;9:1046636.

254. Ruiz D, Haynes C, Marable J, et al. Development of OX40 agonists for canine cancer immunotherapy. iScience 2022;25:105158.

255. Qiu J, Yang Y, Kong J, et al. Quantification of pharmacokinetic profiles of a recombinant canine PD-1 fusion protein by validated sandwich ELISA method. Front Vet Sci 2022;9:951176.

256. Atherton MJ, Rotolo A, Haran KP, et al. Case Report: Clinical and Serological Hallmarks of Cytokine Release Syndrome in a Canine B Cell Lymphoma Patient Treated With Autologous CAR-T Cells. Front Vet Sci 2022;9:824982.

257. Igase M, Inanaga S, Tani K, et al. Long-term survival of dogs with stage 4 oral malignant melanoma treated with anti-canine PD-1 therapeutic antibody: A follow-up case report. Vet Comp Oncol 2022;20:901–5.

258. Sakai O, Yamamoto H, Igase M, et al. Optimization of Culture Conditions for the Generation of Canine CD20-CAR-T Cells for Adoptive Immunotherapy. In Vivo 2022;36:764–72.

259. Boss MK, Watts R, Harrison LG, et al. Immunologic Effects of Stereotactic Body Radiotherapy in Dogs with Spontaneous Tumors and the Impact of Intratumoral OX40/TLR Agonist Immunotherapy. Int J Mol Sci 2022;23.

260. Pinard CJ, Hocker SE, Poon AC, et al. Evaluation of PD-1 and PD-L1 expression in canine urothelial carcinoma cell lines. Vet Immunol Immunopathol 2022;243: 110367.

261. Mason NJ, Chester N, Xiong A, et al. Development of a fully canine anti-canine CTLA4 monoclonal antibody for comparative translational research in dogs with spontaneous tumors. mAbs 2021;13:2004638.

262. Stevenson VB, Perry SN, Todd M, et al. PD-1, PD-L1, and PD-L2 Gene Expression and Tumor Infiltrating Lymphocytes in Canine Melanoma. Vet Pathol 2021; 58:692–8.

263. Cronise KE, Das S, Hernandez BG, et al. Characterizing the molecular and immune landscape of canine bladder cancer. Vet Comp Oncol 2022;20:69–81.

264. Urbano AC, Nascimento C, Soares M, et al. Clinical Relevance of the serum CTLA-4 in Cats with Mammary Carcinoma. Sci Rep 2020;10:3822.

265. Nascimento C, Urbano AC, Gameiro A, et al. Serum PD-1/PD-L1 Levels, Tumor Expression and PD-L1 Somatic Mutations in HER2-Positive and Triple Negative Normal-Like Feline Mammary Carcinoma Subtypes. Cancers 2020;12.

266. Valente S, Nascimento C, Gameiro A, et al. TIM-3 Is a Potential Immune Checkpoint Target in Cats with Mammary Carcinoma. Cancers 2023;15.

267. Maekawa N, Konnai S, Asano Y, et al. Molecular characterization of feline immune checkpoint molecules and establishment of PD-L1 immunohistochemistry for feline tumors. PLoS One 2023;18:e0281143.

268. Nishibori S, Sakurai M, Kagawa Y, et al. Cross-reactivity of anti-human programmed cell death ligand 1 (PD-L1) monoclonal antibody, clone 28-8 against feline PD-L1. J Vet Med Sci 2023;85:592–600.

269. Chambers MR, Bentley RT, Crossman DK, et al. The One Health Consortium: Design of a Phase I Clinical Trial to Evaluate M032, a Genetically Engineered HSV-1 Expressing IL-12, in Combination With a Checkpoint Inhibitor in Canine Patients With Sporadic High Grade Gliomas. Front Surg 2020;7:59.

270. Porcellato I, Brachelente C, Cappelli K, et al. FoxP3, CTLA-4, and IDO in Canine Melanocytic Tumors. Vet Pathol 2021;58:42–52.

271. Igase M, Nemoto Y, Itamoto K, et al. A pilot clinical study of the therapeutic antibody against canine PD-1 for advanced spontaneous cancers in dogs. Sci Rep 2020;10:18311.

272. Ganbaatar O, Konnai S, Okagawa T, et al. PD-L1 expression in equine malignant melanoma and functional effects of PD-L1 blockade. PLoS One 2020;15: e0234218.

273. Maekawa N, Konnai S, Nishimura M, et al. PD-L1 immunohistochemistry for canine cancers and clinical benefit of anti-PD-L1 antibody in dogs with pulmonary metastatic oral malignant melanoma. npj Precis Oncol 2021;5:10.

274. Pantelyushin S, Ranninger E, Guerrera D, et al. Cross-reactivity and functionality of approved human immune checkpoint blockers in dogs. Cancers 2021;13.

275. Heinzerling L, Goldinger SM. A review of serious adverse effects under treatment with checkpoint inhibitors. Curr Opin Oncol 2017;29:136–44.

276. Kumar V, Chaudhary N, Garg M, et al. Current Diagnosis and Management of Immune Related Adverse Events (irAEs) Induced by Immune Checkpoint Inhibitor Therapy. Front Pharmacol 2017;8:49.

277. Abe S, Nagata H, Crosby EJ, et al. Combination of ultrasound-based mechanical disruption of tumor with immune checkpoint blockade modifies tumor microenvironment and augments systemic antitumor immunity. J Immunother Cancer 2022;10.

278. Tang R, He H, Lin X, et al. Novel combination strategy of high intensity focused ultrasound (HIFU) and checkpoint blockade boosted by bioinspired and oxygen-supplied nanoprobe for multimodal imaging-guided cancer therapy. J Immunother Cancer 2023;11.

279. Wu Q, Xia Y, Xiong X, et al. Focused ultrasound-mediated small-molecule delivery to potentiate immune checkpoint blockade in solid tumors. Front Pharmacol 2023;14:1169608.

280. Castelló CM, de Carvalho MT, Bakuzis AF, et al. Local tumour nanoparticle thermal therapy: A promising immunomodulatory treatment for canine cancer. Vet Comp Oncol 2022;20:752–66.

281. Ryu MO, Lee SH, Ahn JO, et al. Treatment of solid tumors in dogs using veterinary high-intensity focused ultrasound: A retrospective clinical study. Vet J 2018;234:126–9.

282. Horise Y, Maeda M, Konishi Y, et al. Sonodynamic Therapy With Anticancer Micelles and High-Intensity Focused Ultrasound in Treatment of Canine Cancer. Front Pharmacol 2019;10:545.

283. Carroll J, Coutermarsh-Ott S, Klahn SL, et al. High intensity focused ultrasound for the treatment of solid tumors: a pilot study in canine cancer patients. Int J Hyperther 2022;39:855–64.

284. Ashar H, Singh A, Kishore D, et al. Enabling Chemo-Immunotherapy with HIFU in Canine Cancer Patients. Ann Biomed Eng 2023. https://doi.org/10.1007/s10439-023-03194-1.

285. LeBlanc AK, Breen M, Choyke P, et al. Perspectives from man's best friend: National Academy of Medicine's Workshop on Comparative Oncology. Sci Transl Med 2016;8:324ps325.

286. Khanna C, Lindblad-Toh K, Vail D, et al. The dog as a cancer model. Nat Biotechnol 2006;24:1065–6.

287. Khanna C, London C, Vail D, et al. Guiding the optimal translation of new cancer treatments from canine to human cancer patients. Clin Cancer Res 2009;15: 5671–7.
288. Paoloni M, Khanna C. Translation of new cancer treatments from pet dogs to humans. Nat Rev Cancer 2008;8:147–56.
289. Gordon I, Paoloni M, Mazcko C, et al. The Comparative Oncology Trials Consortium: using spontaneously occurring cancers in dogs to inform the cancer drug development pathway. PLoS Med 2009;6:e1000161.
290. Ranieri G, Gadaleta CD, Patruno R, et al. A model of study for human cancer: Spontaneous occurring tumors in dogs. Biological features and translation for new anticancer therapies. Crit Rev Oncol Hematol 2013;88:187–97.
291. Angstadt AY, Thayanithy V, Subramanian S, et al. A genome-wide approach to comparative oncology: high-resolution oligonucleotide aCGH of canine and human osteosarcoma pinpoints shared microaberrations. Cancer Genet 2012;205: 572–87.
292. LeBlanc AK, Mazcko C, Brown DE, et al. Creation of an NCI comparative brain tumor consortium: informing the translation of new knowledge from canine to human brain tumor patients. Neuro Oncol 2016;18:1209–18.
293. Seelig DM, Avery AC, Ehrhart EJ, et al. The Comparative Diagnostic Features of Canine and Human Lymphoma. Vet Sci 2016;3.
294. Fulkerson CM, Dhawan D, Ratliff TL, et al. Naturally Occurring Canine Invasive Urinary Bladder Cancer: A Complementary Animal Model to Improve the Success Rate in Human Clinical Trials of New Cancer Drugs. Int J Genomics 2017;2017:6589529.
295. Von Rueden SK, Fan TM. Cancer-Immunity Cycle and Therapeutic Interventions- Opportunities for Including Pet Dogs With Cancer. Front Oncol 2021;11: 773420.

New Therapies in Veterinary Oncology

Christine Mullin, VMD[a], Craig A. Clifford, DVM, MS[a,*],
Chad M. Johannes, DVM[b]

KEYWORDS

- Laverdia • Canalevia • Stelfonta • Novel therapy

KEY POINTS

- Laverdia-CA1 (verdinexor tablets) is the first oral drug for dogs with lymphoma (LSA) and has demonstrated efficacy as a single-agent treatment for all types of canine LSA.
- Canalevia-CA1 (crofelemer delayed-release tablets) is the first conditionally approved oral drug for dogs with chemotherapy-induced diarrhea.
- Stelfonta (tigilanol tiglate injection) is the first Food and Drug Administration-approved intratumoral therapy for local control of canine mast cell tumors. A complete response rate of 75% following one injection/treatment was noted in the pivotal trial.

LAVERDIA-CA1 (VERDINEXOR)

Introduction

Despite far-reaching and diligent research efforts aimed at improving the outcomes of dogs with lymphoma (LSA), the overall prognosis for this cancer has remained unchanged for more than 30 years. Therefore, the identification of novel therapeutic targets and the development of corresponding therapies is critical to the advancement of canine LSA treatment.

Laverdia-CA1 (verdinexor tablets) is the first oral drug for dogs with LSA and was conditionally approved (CA) by the Food and Drug Administration (FDA) in 2021, pending a full demonstration of effectiveness. Conditional approval allows veterinarians to obtain and use Laverdia-CA1 as the company continues clinical trials to support full approval. Verdinexor is a small molecule inhibitor, specifically a selective inhibitor of nuclear transport (SINE) drug. Verdinexor targets exportin-1 (XPO1)—a transport protein overexpressed in certain types of cancer, including LSA. XPO1 exports tumor suppressor proteins (TSPs) from the nuclei of cells, thus leaving the cell vulnerable to uncontrolled cell growth and proliferation. Verdinexor binds to XPO1, trapping TSPs inside the nucleus, thus triggering programmed cell death of LSA cells while sparing normal cells.[1–3]

[a] BluePearl Pet Hospital – Malvern, 40 Three Tun Road, Malvern, PA 19355, USA; [b] Colorado State University, 300 West Drake Road, Fort Collins, CO 80526, USA
* Corresponding author.
E-mail address: Craig.clifford@bluepearlvet.com

Vet Clin Small Anim 54 (2024) 469–476
https://doi.org/10.1016/j.cvsm.2023.12.003
0195-5616/24/© 2023 Elsevier Inc. All rights reserved.

Current Evidence

Verdinexor has demonstrated efficacy as a single-agent treatment for all types of canine LSA—B-cell, T-cell, naïve, and first relapse following either a single or multi-agent protocol. In a phase II study, the objective response rate (partial response or CR) was 34.5% (20/58 dogs). For patients with naïve B-cell LSA, the overall response rate was 57%, whereas it was 43% for relapsed B-cell LSA. For T-cell LSA, traditionally more refractory to current treatment protocols than B-cell LSA, verdinexor demonstrated clinical benefit in 71% of the dogs, whether naïve or relapse. The median time to progression (ie, duration of response) was 36.5 days (range 7–244) for naïve patients and 22 days (range 7–194) for relapsed patients. The clinical benefit rate (CR + partial response + stable disease) across both naïve and relapsed B-cell and T-cell cases was 55%, with a median duration of benefit of 71 days (range 21–273 days).[2,3]

Most adverse effects of verdinexor are mild but may include lethargy, anorexia, weight loss, vomiting, diarrhea, polyuria, polydipsia, elevated liver enzymes, and thrombocytopenia.[1,2] Side effects are typically manageable with supportive care and medications to address anorexia and other gastrointestinal signs, modulation of verdinexor dose, and administration of low-dose prednisone.[1–3]

Discussion

Verdinexor has been shown not to be a substrate for P-glycoprotein and therefore should not be subject to multi-drug resistance.[4] In addition, there is no evidence to date suggesting that SINE class drugs increase the expression of P glycoprotein and initiate MDR. These two differences from corticosteroids (ie, prednisone) suggest that verdinexor could be a useful first-line therapy for dogs recently diagnosed with LSA both in the interim before initiating a chemotherapy protocol without concern about having a negative impact, and as a single-agent targeted therapy if referral for traditional chemotherapy is declined.[4] Additional studies are underway to help better understand the ideal role for verdinexor in the treatment of canine LSAs.

Aside from canine LSA, verdinexor has also shown in vitro activity against canine osteosarcoma cell lines, canine melanoma cell lines, canine mammary carcinoma cell lines, and canine transitional cell carcinoma cell lines, at physiologically relevant doses.[5–7] As such, ongoing research as to the utility of verdinexor will likely also include investigation of its value as an agent against solid tumors.

Summary

Pending additional data, these authors see several scenarios where verdinexor may be incorporated into clinical practice for management of canine LSA, including.

- Pet owner declines referral but wants to do more than prednisone alone.
- As a palliative care option for dogs whose disease is prednisone-resistant or for those that cannot receive prednisone.
- Patient is to be seen by a specialist, but referral appointment is several weeks away.
- Patient has failed standard-of-care chemotherapy and owner declines other rescue chemotherapy protocols.
- As a maintenance therapy after traditional chemotherapy for a patient with poor indicators and perceived high risk for early relapse.
- For patients with unique presentations of lymphoma including epitheliotropic LSAs and indolent LSAs, particularly if traditional chemotherapy has failed or is declined.

Clinics Care Points

- Laverdia-CA1 can used for any type of canine LSA (the label is broad).
- Laverdia-CA1 is commercially available in three tablets sizes: 2.5 mg, 10 mg, and 50 mg.

The recommended starting dose is 1.25 mg/kg twice weekly (every 72 hours), with the option to increase the dose to 1.5 mg/kg twice weekly if well-tolerated.[3] The package insert includes a helpful chart that lists the number of each tablet size that is needed to provide the dose for the different ranges of canine body weights.

- Laverdia-CA1 should be given to dogs immediately after eating, as this increases the amount of drug absorbed into the bloodstream.
- Approved chemotherapy gloves should be worn when handling Laverdia-CA1 and cleaning up excrement of a dog undergoing treatment with Laverdia-CA1.
- Children, those who are pregnant, may become pregnant, or are nursing should not handle Laverdia-CA1 or touch the feces, urine, vomit, or saliva of treated dogs.
- Verdinexor does not seem to induce P-glycoprotein, which has been implicated in chemotherapy resistance and notoriously develops secondary to prednisone administration.

CANALEVIA-CA1 (CROFELEMER DELAYED-RELEASE TABLETS)
Introduction

Chemotherapy has become a mainstay in the treatment of cancer in veterinary medicine. Although the dose intensity in veterinary oncology is lower than in physician-based oncology, it is not without possible side effects. Chemotherapy-induced diarrhea (CID) is a common side effect of dog chemotherapy treatments.[8,9] CID is a complex process. Chemotherapy can target rapidly dividing cells lining the gastrointestinal tract, leading to gastrointestinal toxicity and diarrhea. Chemotherapy is also believed to disrupt the balance of chloride ions and fluid flow into the gastrointestinal (GI) lumen, leading to secretory diarrhea. This can result in damage to gastrointestinal epithelium, damage to the enteric nervous system, and gastrointestinal inflammation. Chloride channels, which control the fluid flow into the intestinal lumen, are a target for remediating CID. CID compromises the physical well-being of dogs and can also impact their psychological health due to discomfort and an altered daily routine. Effective management strategies are therefore essential to mitigate these challenges and ensure successful cancer treatment.

There is no standard of care for CID in veterinary medicine, with metronidazole being the most commonly prescribed drug.[10–14] Several concerns have recently been raised about the widespread use of metronidazole in veterinary medicine.[12–14] First, it is not indicated for use in dogs. Its intended use in humans is as an antiprotozoal and antibacterial.[13] Still, an infectious agent does not cause CID, and the recent emergence of resistant bacteria in both veterinary and human health care facilities has questioned the overuse of metronidazole. Recent studies have shown metronidazole to cause more disruption to the gut flora, where historically, it was thought to provide an anti-inflammatory and flora-balancing effect in the gut.[10,12,14] Metronidazole is associated with several side effects, including nausea/vomiting, diarrhea, drooling, gagging/regurgitation, fatigue, loss of appetite, discoloration of urine, and fever.[10,11]

Current Evidence

Crofelemer, the active in Canalevia-CA1, is a natural botanic drug sustainably harvested from the sap of the South American Croton lechleri tree. It has been approved by the US FDA for treating diarrhea in humans with HIV/AIDS.[15,16]

In humans, crofelemer is an inhibitor of both the cyclic adenosine monophosphate-stimulated cystic fibrosis transmembrane conductance regulator (CFTR) chloride ion (Cl−) channel and the calcium-activated Cl− channels (CaCC) at the luminal membrane of enterocytes.[15,16] The CFTR and CaCC Cl− channels regulate Cl− and the osmotic gradient, which causes fluid influx into the lumen. Crofelemer inhibits the hypersecretion of Cl− in diarrhea and normalizes the fluid influx into the GI tract.[15,16] The mechanism of action in the dog has not been fully characterized.

In December 2021, Canalevia-CA1 (crofelemer delayed-release tablets 125 mg) became the first and only FDA-CA product for treating CID in dogs. Canalevia-CA1 is an antidiarrheal, enteric-coated tablet for oral administration to dogs with CID. It is a canine-specific formulation of crofelemer that acts locally within the GI tract and is minimally absorbed into the bloodstream, providing a well-tolerated and nontoxic drug product. The reasonable expectation of effectiveness of Canalevia-CA1 was established in a study with 24 dogs with acute diarrhea (12 active and 12 control dogs) receiving treatment orally twice daily more than 72 hours. At 72 hours, 9 of 12 dogs (75%) in the active group were treatment successes compared with 3 of 12 dogs (25%) in the control group.[17] The dose of Canalevia-CA1 is one tablet orally twice daily for 3 days for dogs weighing ≤ 140 pounds and two tablets orally twice daily for dogs weighing greater than 140 pounds. Canalevia-CA1 can be given with or without food and is very safe, with no significant toxicity noted in safety studies where dogs received up to 10× the recommended dose. Freedom of information summary: Infectious etiologies of diarrhea should be ruled out before using Canalevia-CA1, and it should not be used for hemorrhagic diarrhea under its current conditional label.

Summary

CID poses a significant challenge in the management of cancer in dogs. Canalevia, with its novel mechanism of action and proven efficacy in managing diarrhea in other contexts, offers a potential treatment option for CID. Further research, including larger clinical trials and long-term studies, is warranted to establish its safety, optimal dosing, and long-term benefits in this patient population.

Clinics Care Points

- CID is a challenging adverse event associated with many chemotherapeutics, and before Canalevia -CA1, no approved drugs were available for its treatment.
- CID is not a result of a bacterial infection and with the growing concern over the inappropriate use of antimicrobials, alternatives options are needed.
- Canalevia-CA1 is a natural botanic drug sustainably harvested from the sap of the South American Croton lechleri tree and is the first conditionally approved oral drug for dogs with CID.
- Canalevia-CA1 has a novel mechanism of actions and acts locally in the gastrointestinal tract.
- The labeled dose is one tablet orally twice daily for 3 days for dogs weighing ≤ 140 pounds and two orally twice daily for dogs weighing greater than 140 pounds (Canalevia-CA1 package insert).

STELFONTA (TIGILANOL TIGLATE INJECTION)
Introduction

Surgical excision is the mainstay for local control of canine mast cell tumors (MCT) yet surgery is not an option for several dogs for a variety of reasons (anatomic location, patient status, anesthetic risk/concern, client decision). The FDA approval of Stelfonta in 2020 provided veterinarians with an effective nonsurgical therapeutic option for local control of canine MCT.[18] Given the novel mechanism of action and unique intratumoral delivery method of Stelfonta, there is a learning curve to clinical incorporation and case management. Becoming comfortable with Stelfonta case selection, treatment delivery, and wound management will provide veterinarians with an effective local treatment alternative for canine MCT cases where surgery is not ideal.[19]

Current Evidence

Stelfonta (tigilanol tiglate) is a novel diterpene ester derived from the seeds of the native Australian blushwood tree (*Fontainea picrosperma*). It is a potent cellular signaling molecule with a multifactorial mode of action.[18,19] The antitumor effect of tigilanol tiglate is due to three primary mechanisms.

1. Direct oncolysis of tumor cells due to disruption of mitochondrial function
2. Protein kinase C activation causing an acute inflammatory response resulting in local tumor hypoxia and recruitment of innate immune cells
3. Vascular necrosis resulting from destruction of tumor vasculature (which is more sensitive to the effects of tigilanol tiglate than is normal tissue vasculature).

By upregulation of key wound repair pathways, tigilanol tiglate promotes re-epithelialization via increased extracellular matrix production and keratinocyte differentiation. Tigilanol tiglate also provides an antimicrobial effect at the tumor wound site. Both of these effects are beneficial in supporting effective wound healing.[20–22]

Stelfonta is indicated for the treatment of non-metastatic cutaneous (located anywhere on the body) or subcutaneous (located at or distal to the elbow or hock) MCT in dogs. Treated MCT should be $\leq$ 10 cm^3 in volume (consult product package insert for calculation formula and dosing guidelines).[18]

The registrational trial that provided safety and efficacy data for the approval of Stelfonta enrolled 123 dogs with MCT (81 treated with Stelfonta, 42 untreated controls) in a primary care setting. Response was evaluated at 28 days posttreatment. Single treatment with Stelfonta resulted in a CR of 75% compared with 5% in the control group. For those dogs that did not achieve a CR with the first treatment, a second treatment improved the overall CR to 88%. The study followed dogs for a total of 84 days posttreatment. No MCT recurrence was observed in 93% of dogs that responded to Stelfonta treatment.[19] Most of the wound sites were healed within 28 to 42 days following treatment and only rarely required bandaging or antimicrobial therapy.[22] The most common adverse effects noted in this study were directly related to the mechanism of action of tigilanol tiglate and included wound formation, injection site pain, lameness in the treated limb, and injection site bruising and erythema. Additional side effects were generally low grade and transient, including vomiting, diarrhea, hypoalbuminemia, and anorexia.[19]

A subsequent publication reporting on a subset of these dogs where follow-up was available showed that 89% of responding dogs demonstrated no local recurrence 12 months following Stelfonta treatment. The 11% that experienced local recurrence did so within the first 6 months following treatment.[23] An additional publication reported outcomes for the dogs in this study combined with dogs from Australian studies with cytologically diagnosed high-grade MCT. Within this group of dogs, 56% of those with high-grade MCT achieved and maintained CR at 84 days following one or two treatments with Stelfonta.[24]

Clinical use of Stelfonta in the treatment of multiple synchronous canine MCT has been described. The study reported on 9 dogs with a total of 32 MCT treated.

Evaluation of the individual tumors at 28 days posttreatment indicated a CR in 81%. Of the 22 tumors evaluable at 6 months posttreatment, no MCT recurrence was observed.[25]

Stelfonta may provide a local treatment option for other solid tumors in dogs, but safety and efficacy data in those tumors are anecdotal at this time. Clinical trials evaluating Stelfonta for treatment of canine soft tissue sarcoma are ongoing. The initial clinical efficacy of Stelfonta in two horses (fibroblastic sarcoid, squamous cell carcinoma) has also been reported.[26] Additional clinical trials evaluating Stelfonta for treatment of equine sarcoid and melanoma are ongoing.

Summary

Stelfonta provides a novel mechanism of action and high single-treatment efficacy rate for local control of canine MCT. It should be considered for local therapy of MCT in dogs, factoring in the size and anatomic location of the tumor, overall patient status, any anesthetic concerns, and client preference. Appropriate case selection and client education is important when considering Stelfonta. Clients should have a good understanding and appropriate expectations regarding wound formation and management to help ensure best treatment outcomes. Given the novel treatment delivery route and wound management intricacies, veterinarians should not hesitate to contact their regional oncologist, colleagues with Stelfonta treatment experience, or the manufacturer (Virbac) for case selection and management guidance.

CLINICS CARE POINTS

- Concomitant medication (prednisone/prednisolone, H1-blocker, H2-blocker) dosing and timing should be strictly followed per the package insert to decrease the potential for systemic signs caused by mast cell degranulation.
- MCT volume measurements and dosing calculations outlined in the package insert should be followed closely and double-checked before treatment.
- Stelfonta is administered as an intratumoral injection via a 23-gauge needle. Use a single injection site and a fanning motion to distribute drug throughout the tumor. Sedation may be needed for administration.
- Pain control medications should be considered for 5 to 7 days following treatment.
- The wound created by Stelfonta treatment should be allowed to heal without bandaging, debridement, or antimicrobial therapy (rare exceptions do occur).
- If CR is not noted following initial treatment with Stelfonta, retreatment is possible. Wait at least 28 days following the most recent Stelfonta treatment before repeated dosing at the same site.
- As histologic grade is not available for MCT treated with Stelfonta, consideration of other prognostic factors (including cytologic grade and regional lymph node aspiration/cytology for metastasis evaluation) is important. If incisional biopsy is performed on the MCT before Stelfonta treatment, allow the site to heal for 14 days to prevent leakage of Stelfonta at the time of administration.
- The efficacy and safety of Stelfonta used in combination with other treatment modalities (chemotherapy, radiation therapy, immunotherapy) for canine MCT is currently not well-defined. A veterinary oncologist should be consulted for discussion of options on an individual case basis.

DISCLOSURE

C. Mullin: No disclosures to report. C.A. Clifford: Speaker, advisory board member and consultant with Jaguar Animal Health and Anivive. C.M. Johannes: Speaker, advisory board member and consultant with QBiotics Group; advisory board member with Jaguar Animal Health.

REFERENCES

1. London CA, Bernabe LF, Barnard S, et al. Preclinical evaluation of the novel, orally bioavailable Selective Inhibitor of Nuclear Export (SINE) KPT-335 in spontaneous canine cancer: results of a phase I study. PLoS One 2014;9(2):e87585.
2. Sadowski AR, Gardner HL, Borgatti A, et al. Phase II study of the oral selective inhibitor of nuclear export (SINE) KPT-335 (verdinexor) in dogs with lymphoma. BMC Vet Res 2018;14(1):250.
3. Laverdia-CA1 Package Insert, Anivive Lifesciences, 2020.
4. Mealey KL, Burke NS. Assessment of verdinexor as a canine P-glycoprotein substrate. J Vet Pharmacol Ther 2023;46(4):264–7.
5. Breit MN, Kisseberth WC, Bear MD, et al. Biologic activity of the novel orally bioavailable selective inhibitor of nuclear export (SINE) KPT-335 against canine melanoma cell lines. BMC Vet Res 2014;10:160.
6. Breitbach JT, Louke DS, Tobin SJ, et al. The selective inhibitor of nuclear export (SINE) verdinexor exhibits biologic activity against canine osteosarcoma cell lines. Vet Comp Oncol 2012;19(2):362–73.
7. Grayton JE, Miller T, Wilson-Robles H. In vitro evaluation of Selective Inhibitors of Nuclear Export (SINE) drugs KPT-185 and KPT-335 against canine mammary carcinoma and transitional cell carcinoma tumor initiating cells. Vet Comp Oncol 2017;15(4):1455–67.
8. Vail DM. Supporting the Veterinary Cancer Patient on Chemotherapy: Neutropenia and Gastrointestinal Toxicity. Top Companion Anim Med 2009;24:122–9.
9. MacDonald V. Chemotherapy: managing side effects and safe handling. The Canadian Veterinary Journal = La Revue Vétérinaire Canadienne 2009;50:665–8.
10. Fitzgerald KT, Metronidazole. In: Talcott PA, Peterson ME, editors. Small animal toxicology, 3rd edition, 2013, Saunders Elsevier; St Louis (MO), 653–658.
11. Lee JA. Metronidazole Risks. Plumb's Therapeutics Brief 2014;10–1.
12. Palma E, Tilocco B, Rocando P. Antimicrobial Resistance in Veterinary Medicine: An Overview. Int J Mol Sci 2020;21(6):1914.
13. Ceruelos AH, Romero-Quezada LC, Ruvalcaba JC, et al. Therapeutic uses of metronidazole and its side effects: an update. Eur Rev Med Pharmacol Sci 2019;23(397):401.
14. Igarashi H, Maeda S, Ohno K, et al. Effect of Oral Administration of Metronidazole or Prednisolone on Fecal Microbiota in Dogs 2015; doi:10.1371/journal.pone.0107909.
15. Cottreau J, Tucker A, Crutchley R, et al. Crofelemer for the treatment of secretory diarrhea. Expet Rev Gastroenterol Hepatol 2012;6:17–23.
16. Frampton JE. Crofelemer: A Review of its Use in the Management of Non-Infectious Diarrhoea in Adult Patients with HIV/AIDS on Antiretroviral Therapy. Drugs 2013;73:1121–9.
17. FREEDOM OF INFORMATION SUMMARY: APPLICATION FOR CONDITIONAL APPROVAL. Application Number 141-552. CANALEVIA™-CA1. Pg 1-27.
18. Stelfonta Package Insert, Virbac, 2020.

19. De Ridder TR, Campbell JE, Burke-Schwarz C, et al. Randomized controlled clinical study evaluating the efficacy and safety of intratumoral treatment of canine mast cell tumors with tigilanol tiglate (EBC-46). J Vet Intern Med 2021;35(1): 415–29.

20. Moses RL, Boyle GM, Howard-Jones RA, et al. Novel epoxy-tiglianes stimulate skin keratinocyte wound healing responses and re-epithelialization via protein kinase C activation. Biochem Pharmacol 2020;178:114048.

21. Powell LC, Cullen JK, Boyle GM, et al. Topical, immunomodulatory epoxy-tiglianes induce biofilm disruption and healing in acute and chronic skin wounds. Sci Transl Med 2022;14(662):eabn3758.

22. Reddell P, De Ridder TR, Morton JM, et al. Wound formation, wound size, and progression of wound healing after intratumoral treatment of mast cell tumors in dogs with tigilanol tiglate. J Vet Intern Med 2021;35(1):430–41.

23. Jones PD, Campbell JE, Brown G, et al. Recurrence-free interval 12 months after local treatment of mast cell tumors in dogs using intratumoral injection of tigilanol tiglate. J Vet Intern Med 2021;35(1):451–5.

24. Brown GK, Campbell JE, Jones PD, et al. Intratumoral treatment of 18 cytologically diagnosed canine high-grade mast cell tumours with tigilanol tiglate. Front Vet Sci 2021;8:675804.

25. Brown GK, Finlay JR, Straw RC, et al. Treatment of multiple synchronous canine mast cell tumors using intratumoral tigilanol tiglate. Front Vet Sci 2022;9:1003165.

26. De Ridder T, Ruppin M, Wheeless M, et al. Use of the intratumoral anticancer drug tigilanol tiglate in two horses. Front Vet Sci 2020;7:639.

Novel Treatments for Lymphoma

Douglas H. Thamm, VMD, DACVIM (Oncology)

KEYWORDS

- Chemotherapy • Canine • Feline • Cancer

KEY POINTS

- Conventional cyclophosphamide, hydroxydaunorubicin, Oncovin, prednisone (CHOP)–based chemotherapy results in high response rates in dogs, but the vast majority of dogs will eventually relapse.
- Response rates to CHOP-based chemotherapy are lower in cats with intermediate-grade to high-grade lymphoma than in dogs, but low-grade small-cell lymphoma, which has a more favorable outcome with conservative treatment, is more common.
- A variety of alterations in conventional CHOP-based protocols, such as omission of asparaginase or corticosteroids and substituting oral for injectable cyclophosphamide, can be employed in dogs with lymphoma without impact on efficacy.
- There are multiple chemotherapy protocols that have been evaluated for treatment of relapsed/refractory canine lymphoma. There is no optimal protocol, but in general, multi-agent protocols appear superior to single drugs.
- The novel small molecules verdinexor (Laverdia-CA1) and rabacfosadine succinate (Tanovea) have demonstrated meaningful antitumor activity and reasonable safety in dogs with lymphoma, leading to conditional (verdinexor) or full (rabacfosadine) approval by the Food and Drug Administration-Center for Veterinary Medicine (FDA-CVM) for the treatment of canine lymphoma.

INTRODUCTION

Lymphoma is one of the most common neoplastic diseases in companion animals. While conventional chemotherapy has the potential to induce remission and prolong life, relapse is common and novel approaches are needed to improve outcome. This review will cover the basics of canine and feline lymphoma treatment, options for treatment of relapsed/refractory disease, and recent advances in standard of care therapy as well as new treatments that are in varying stages of regulatory approval.

Flint Animal Cancer Center, College of Veterinary Medicine and Biomedical Sciences, Colorado State University, 300 West Drake Road, Fort Collins, CO 80523-1620 USA
E-mail address: dthamm@colostate.edu

Vet Clin Small Anim 54 (2024) 477–490
https://doi.org/10.1016/j.cvsm.2023.12.004
0195-5616/24/© 2023 Elsevier Inc. All rights reserved.

REVIEW OF CONVENTIONAL TREATMENTS FOR LYMPHOMA
Canine Lymphoma

Owing to lymphoma's systemic presentation, chemotherapy is the mainstay of treatment. A large number of single-agent and multi-agent chemotherapy protocols have been investigated over the last 40 years; however, 1 optimal chemotherapy protocol has not been identified that integrates positive outcome, toxicity, and cost.

Corticosteroids alone have been shown to induce at least partial remission in many dogs and cats with lymphoma by their direct cytotoxic effect, as well as being associated with symptomatic improvement. Oral corticosteroids (most commonly prednisone/prednisolone at 2 mg/kg/day by mouth initially, then tapered over 1–3 weeks to 0.5–1 mg/kg/day) are a reasonable treatment for some owners if chemotherapy is declined. While most patients will experience meaningful short-term improvement, the reported median survival time (MST) was 50 days in 1 recent report,[1] and corticosteroids appear to induce chemotherapy resistance; thus, attempting chemotherapy after prednisone has failed, while not impossible, may be considerably less successful than in a patient that has not been pretreated.

A relatively simple, inexpensive chemotherapy protocol with intermediate efficacy is single-agent doxorubicin (DOX). This is reasonably affordable since DOX is available in generic form, and requires only 1 injection every 3 weeks. Approximately 65% to 85% of dogs will respond to single-agent DOX, with reported median response durations (MRDs) of 100 to 170 days.[2–5] Two unique adverse effects (AEs) of DOX are its potential for cumulative cardiac toxicity in dogs and its potential to cause severe skin necrosis if extravasated.

Generally, the most successful chemotherapy protocols are multi-agent protocols that include DOX. These protocols, referred to generically as cyclophosphamide (CYC), hydroxydaunorubicin (doxorubicin hydrochloride [DOX]), Oncovin (vincristine [VCR]), prednisone (CHOP)–based protocols, are employed by many oncologists and utilize sequential injections of VCR, CYC, and DOX, combined with daily prednisone for the first 4 weeks. Published CHOP-based protocols generally range from 15 to 25 weeks in duration (**Table 1**). Complete response (CR) rates are 85% to 95%, median progression free-survival (MPFS) times are 5 to 9 months, and MSTs are approximately 12 months, with 20% to 25% of dogs living up to 2 years.[6–11] Unfortunately, all but approximately 5% of patients will eventually relapse.

Most current CHOP protocols suspend therapy following 4 to 6 months of treatment: monthly rechecks are then pursued to assess remission status. A recent study confirmed an apparent lack of benefit to "maintenance" therapy following completion of this initial period of intensive treatment.[12]

Factors that historically have carried the most prognostic significance for remission duration and survival include clinical signs at presentation (substage b), hypercalcemia, mediastinal lymphadenopathy, and significant bone marrow infiltration or circulating atypical lymphocytes.[13–15] Both hypercalcemia and mediastinal lymphadenopathy are likely surrogates for lymphomas with a T cell immunophenotype, a powerful predictor of outcome. Most veterinary pathology laboratories are capable of immunophenotyping lymphomas through immunohistochemistry. Immunophenotyping alternatively can be performed on fine-needle aspirates using immunocytochemistry, via flow cytometry, or via polymerase chain reaction for antigen receptor rearrangement.[16–18]

Feline Lymphoma

The basic tenets of treatment for feline intermediate-grade to high-grade lymphoma are very similar to canine. One important difference is that single-agent DOX appears

Table 1
Select published cyclophosphamide, hydroxydaunorubicin, oncovin, prednisone (CHOP)–based chemotherapy protocols for canine lymphoma

"UW-25" Protocol

	Week															
	1	2	3	4	6	7	8	9	11	13	15	17	19	21	23	25
Vincristine 0.7 mg/m² IV	*		*		*		*	*	*		*		*		*	
Cyclophosphamide 250 mg/m² PO or IV		*				*				*				*		
Doxorubicin 30 mg/m² IV*				*				*				*				*
Prednisone (mg/kg/day) PO	2	1.5	1	0.5	Discontinue											

"UW-19" Protocol

	Week															
	1	2	3	4	6	7	8	9	11	12	13	14	16	17	18	19
Vincristine 0.7 mg/m² IV	*		*		*		*	*	*		*		*		*	
Cyclophosphamide 250 mg/m² PO or IV		*				*				*				*		
Doxorubicin 30 mg/m² IV*				*				*				*				*
Prednisone (mg/kg/day) PO	2	1.5	1	0.5	Discontinue											

15-wk CHOP Protocol

	Week											
	1	2	3	5	6	7	9	10	11	13	14	15
Vincristine 0.7 mg/m² IV	*		*			*	*			*		
Cyclophosphamide 250 mg/m² PO or IV		*			*			*			*	
Doxorubicin 30 mg/m² IV*				*					*			*
Prednisone (mg/kg/day) PO	2	1.5	1	0.5	Discontinue							

*Doxorubicin is often administered at a dose of 1 mg/kg in dogs weighing less than 15 kg.
Abbreviations: CHOP, cyclophosphamide, hydroxydaunorubicin, Oncovin, prednisone; IV, intravenous; PO, by mouth.
Data from Refs.[7–9,11]

to have substantially less activity in cats.[19,20] Even with CHOP-based chemotherapy, outcomes are generally poorer in cats, with approximately 40% to 45% of cats achieving a CR and approximately 25% experiencing a partial response (PR). Median CR durations are 200 to 400 days and median PR durations are approximately 80 days.[21,22]

In contrast to intermediate-grade to high-grade disease, the majority of cats with low-grade, small-cell gastrointestinal (GI) lymphoma may respond favorably and experience MSTs in the 2 to 3 year range when a protocol employing oral chlorambucil and prednisone is employed. Three different chlorambucil dosing strategies have been reported: 7 mg/m^2 by mouth daily for 5 days repeated every 3 weeks, 20 mg/m^2 by mouth once every 2 weeks, and 2 mg/cat by mouth every 2 to 3 days continuously.[23–25] Importantly, a designation of low-grade, small-cell lymphoma can only be made histologically.

Relapsed/Refractory Disease

Unfortunately, all but approximately 5% of animals with lymphoma will eventually relapse after conventional first-line therapy. When remission is lost following CHOP treatment after an interval with no chemotherapy, many patients may experience a second remission simply by resuming CHOP. However, a rule of thumb is that the second remission is likely to be approximately half as long as the first, and the benefit to CHOP reinduction appears limited in patients that relapse within 2 to 3 months of CHOP completion.[26] At some point, tumor cells will acquire resistance to the initial drugs utilized, and "rescue" or "salvage" chemotherapy drugs or protocols can be considered. A summary of rescue agents/protocols that have been evaluated in dogs is provided in **Table 2**.

While there are many different drugs/protocols that can be utilized in this setting, no 1 agent or protocol is uniformly superior over the others in terms of response rate and duration. Choice of rescue therapy can be influenced by cost, number/frequency of visits, and drug availability, as well as efficacy data. As a group, response rates tend to be higher for multi-agent protocols than for single-agent protocols, although the average response duration remains in the 2 to 3 month range for both types of protocol. Sometimes, attaining a second or third remission can be a matter of trial and error, until an efficacious drug or protocol is found. It is important to counsel owners that there tends to be a "law of diminishing returns" with sequential rescue attempts, meaning that the likelihood of observing a robust response tends to reduce the more agents have been previously utilized.

There is considerably less information available regarding rescue therapy options for cats with lymphoma. Oral CYC appears to be a useful rescue agent in cats with low-grade, small-cell lymphoma that have failed chlorambucil.[60] Rescue protocols that have been evaluated for intermediate-grade to high-grade lymphoma include lomustine methotrexate and cytarabine, mechlorethamine/VCR/procarbazine/prednisone, dexamethasone/melphalan/actinomycin D/cytarabine, and single-agent lomustine.[61–64]

NEWER DATA WITH CONVENTIONAL DRUGS
Asparaginase Versus No Asparaginase

Older publications routinely included a single injection of asparaginase at the beginning of multi-agent treatment; however, 2 studies have demonstrated no improvement in any measure of outcome in dogs receiving asparaginase.[9,65] For this reason, the author chooses to omit asparaginase from initial treatment and save it for potential rescue therapy.

Table 2
Published rescue protocols for canine lymphoma

Drug/Protocol	N	ORR %	CR%	Response Duration	CR Duration	PR Duration	Refs
Mitoxantrone	15–34	21–47	26–47	84	126	42	[27–29]
Actinomycin D	25–49	0-41	0-41	129	129	NR	[30,31]
Lomustine	37–43	26–62	NR/7	15–86	NR/86	NR	[32,33]
Dacarbazine	40	35	2.3	43	144	49	[34]
Rabacfosadine	21–59	56–74	41–48	99–172	168–203	NR	[35–37]
Vinblastine	39	25	8	26.5	NR	NR	[38]
Melphalan	19	16	0	24	N/A	24	[39]
Temozolomide	25	32	4	NR	NR	NR	[40]
Doxorubicin/dacarbazine	15	74	47	NR	NR	NR	[41]
Rabacfosadine/asparaginase	52	69	41	85	144	59	[42]
Asparaginase/lomustine	31–48	87–88	52–65	63–70	90–111	42–54	[43,44]
Temozolomide/anthracycline	18	72	50	40	NR	NR	[45]
Temozolomide/doxorubicin	10	60	10	NR	NR	NR	[40]
Dacarbazine/anthracycline	35	71	62	50	NR	NR	[45]
Lomustine/dacarbazine	57	35	23	NR	83	25	[46]
Carboplatin/cytarabine	14	29	NR	56	NR	NR	[47]
Bleomycin/cytarabine	19	37	0	15	N/A	15	[48]
Mitoxantrone/dacarbazine	44	34	18	97	123	56	[49]
PCP	44	68	41	NR	115	61	[50]
LPP	41	61	29	NR	84	58	[51]
MOPP	117	65	31	NR	63	47	[52]
MVPP	36	25	8	NR	NR	NR	[53]
DMAC	54–100	35–72	16–44	NR/61	62–112	32–44	[54–56]
BOPP	14	50	28	NR	129.5	140	[57]
LOPP	33–44	52–61	27–36	NR/98	NR/l12	NR/84.5	[57,58]
MOMP	88	51	12	56	81	49	[59]

Abbreviations: BOPP, BCNU (carmustine)/Oncovin (vincristine)/procarbazine/prednisone; CR, complete response; DMAC, dexamethasone/melphalan/actinomycin D/cytarabine/; LOPP, lomustine/Oncovin (vincristine)/procarbazine/prednisone; LPP, lomustine/procarbazine/predinsone; MOMP, mechlorethamine/Oncovin (vincristine)/melphalan/prednisone; MOPP, mechlorethamine/Oncovin (vincristine)/procarbazine/prednisone; MVPP, mechlorethamine/vinblastine/procarbazine/prednisone; N, number; N/A, not applicable; NR, not reported; ORR, overall response rate; PCP, prednisone/cyclophosphamide/procarbazine; PR, partial response.

Oral Versus Intravenous Cyclophosphamide

Although most of the statistics generated regarding the efficacy of multi-agent lymphoma chemotherapy protocols have utilized injectable CYC, many clinicians substitute oral CYC at the same dose. Pharmacokinetic analysis comparing oral versus injectable CYC in dogs and cats indicates that while there is a significant difference in plasma exposure to the parent drug, exposure to the active metabolite of CYC, 4-hydroxycyclophosphamide, is similar between the 2 routes of administration. This suggests probable equal efficacy at the same doses.[66,67] One advantage to injectable CYC is that the intended dose can be administered with greater precision than can be attained with tablets, especially in cats and smaller dogs.

Prednisone Versus No Prednisone

There are certain patients where corticosteroid therapy may be contraindicated; for example, patients with unregulated hyperadrenocorticism or diabetes mellitus. Two recent randomized trials evaluated CYC-VCR-DOX–based protocols with or without prednisone and found no difference in any measure of outcome, suggesting that corticosteroids may be omitted if necessary for medical considerations.[68,69]

Is There an All-Oral Chemotherapy Protocol that Is Effective for Canine Lymphoma?

Some owners may be uncomfortable with the idea of injectable chemotherapy but may be more agreeable to oral chemotherapy. While education regarding the tolerability of most injectable chemotherapy protocols and the potential for AEs and need for careful monitoring with oral medications may help to sway some owners, an oral protocol is the only acceptable choice in some cases. Oral chemotherapy appears efficacious for 1 very specific form of canine lymphoma: cutaneous T cell lymphoma (CTCL) in dogs (lomustine ± prednisone); approximately 75% to 85% of dogs with CTCL will have at least a PR to lomustine, although the majority of the responses are incomplete and the MRD is only approximately 3 months.[70,71] Dogs diagnosed with low-grade or indolent lymphoma such as T zone lymphoma may respond well to a conservative oral protocol such as prednisone and chlorambucil[72,73]; however, for most intermediate-grade or high-grade multicentric lymphomas in dogs, no efficacious oral protocol has been identified. One study evaluated the efficacy of prednisone and lomustine as first-line therapy for canine multicentric lymphoma and found it to be no better than prednisone alone.[74]

Should Dogs with T Cell Lymphoma be Treated Differently than Dogs with B Cell Lymphoma?

Dogs with intermediate-grade or high-grade T cell lymphoma generally have inferior outcomes when treated with CHOP-based chemotherapy compared to dogs with B cell lymphoma. Beaver and colleagues[75] evaluated initial response to a single dose of DOX in dogs with either B cell or T cell lymphoma and found a significantly lower overall response rate (ORR) in dogs with T cell lymphoma (50% vs 100%). Multiple reports have evaluated so-called "alkylator rich" chemotherapy protocols such as mechlorethamine-VCR-procarbazine-prednisone (MOPP) or lomustine-VCR-procarbazine-prednisone (LOPP). ORRs have ranged from 73% to 97% (64%–90% CR), with MPFS and MST ranging from 175 to 431 days and 237 to 507 days, respectively.[76–78] However, a separate report documented a similarly high ORR (96%) and relatively similar MPFS (146 days) and MST (235 days) in dogs with T cell lymphoma treated with a CHOP-based protocol.[79] Thus, while definitive evidence of a survival advantage is lacking with these alternative protocols, it is possible that they may result in improved outcomes over more conventional CHOP-based chemotherapy for dogs with non-indolent T cell lymphoma.

Lomustine for Feline Lymphoma

Given that single agent DOX appears to be a less effective "middle of the road" chemotherapy protocol for cats with intermediate-grade to high-grade lymphoma, the default for decades has been a COP (cyclophosphamide-vincristine-prednisone) protocol.[80–82] While efficacy is improved over prednisone alone, there is limited cost savings versus CHOP, and the initial induction period of treatment still requires weekly visits. Furthermore, it is often continued longer term than CHOP protocols are. Given these considerations, there has been a search for a less intensive option that still retains some efficacy. Recently, results of a retrospective study investigating lomus-tine and prednisone for the first-line treatment of cats with intermediate-cell to large-cell GI lymphoma was reported.[83] The ORR was 50% (22% CR), with an MRD of approximately 300 days. The overall MST was approximately 100 days.

Vincristine Versus Vinblastine for Feline Lymphoma

Contrary to what is typically observed in dogs, some GI disturbance following VCR administration appears to be common in cats with lymphoma. A recent prospective study evaluated the use of VCR or vinblastine within the context of a COP-based pro-tocol.[80] There was no difference in response rate, progression-free interval (PFI), or survival time between the arms, but the incidence of GI toxicity was significantly lower in cats receiving vinblastine than those receiving VCR (10% vs 44%).

NEW THERAPIES
Bone Marrow/Stem Cell Transplant

One treatment that is commonly used in some forms of human lymphoma and leuke-mia is high-dose chemotherapy and/or whole-body radiation therapy followed by autologous hematopoietic stem-cell (HSC) or bone marrow transplant to "rescue" the patient from fatal myelosuppression. A combination chemotherapy protocol incor-porating high-dose CYC and autologous bone marrow rescue has been evaluated in pilot studies in dogs, with encouraging preliminary results.[84] Several specialty groups have HSC or bone marrow transplant programs for dogs with lymphoma. Early data suggest acceptable tolerability,[85,86] but definitive evidence of efficacy remains lack-ing. Based on human experience, a more profound antitumor effect may be observed following allogeneic, rather than autologous, transplants, owing to the development of a "graft versus tumor" effect. There is an encouraging case series of long-term survival of dogs with high-grade B cell lymphoma following allogeneic transplant[87]; however, broad deployment of this approach is hampered by challenges identifying haplocom-patible donors.

Monoclonal antibodies

Monoclonal antibodies directed against the CD20 antigen expressed on a majority of human B cell lymphomas (eg, rituximab) have changed the standard of care for the treatment of many forms of B-cell malignancy in humans. When combined with stan-dard of care chemotherapy, improvements in outcome are observed in human pa-tients with intermediate-grade to high grade lymphomas without an increase in toxicity.[88–90] In 2014, a canine-specific anti-CD20 antibody received full licensure of through the US Department of Agriculture (USDA) (Canine Lymphoma Monoclonal Antibody, B-cell; Blontress). Unpublished studies performed following USDA approval failed to demonstrate improvements in outcome over dogs receiving conventional therapy alone, and there were concerns regarding the specificity of the antibody, lead-ing to its withdrawal from the market.

A second anti-canine CD20 monoclonal antibody has been developed. This anti-body has shown good binding characteristics to canine CD20 and demonstrates ev-idence of circulating B cell depletion *in vivo* in laboratory dogs, as well as evidence of antitumor activity in a canine lymphoma mouse xenograft model.[91,92] The current development status of this antibody is unknown.

Small molecules

Verdinexor (Laverdia-CA1) is an orally available inhibitor of a protein called exportin-1, which is responsible for the binding and nuclear export of a large variety of important tumor suppressor proteins. A recent phase-II study of verdinexor in dogs with lymphoma reported an ORR of 37% (71% in dogs with T cell lymphoma), with an MRD of 18 days.[93] GI toxicity, including hyporexia, diarrhea, vomiting, and weight loss, were the most commonly observed AEs. Verdinexor has been granted conditional approval for canine lymphoma treatment by the FDA-CVM. Verdinexor is more thoroughly discussed in another monograph in this edition.

In 2021, the FDA-CVM approved rabacfosadine (RAB) succinate (Tanovea) for the treatment of lymphoma in dogs. RAB is a double prodrug of the guanine nucleotide analog 9-(2-phosphonylmethoxyethyl) guanine (PMEG). Rabacfosadine is hydrolyzed intracellularly and subsequently deaminated to PMEG, a potent inhibitor of the major deoxyribonucleic acid polymerases. RAB is given as a 30-minute intravenous infusion once every 3 weeks. Response rates of 50% to 85% are reported depending on the immunophenotype and degree of pretreatment,[35–37,94] and a combination of alternating RAB and DOX resulted in outcomes similar to those obtained with conventional CHOP-based therapy for naïve canine lymphoma: the ORR was 84% (68% CR), and the overall median PFI was 194 days.[95] As with many cytotoxic drugs for lymphoma, improved outcomes are observed in dogs with B cell disease and in less heavily pretreated dogs.[35–37] Activity has also been observed in dogs with CTCL.[96] In addition to GI and hematologic AEs similar to those observed with other cytotoxic agents, a cumulative dermatopathy can occur, and rare, presumed idiosyncratic, delayed pulmonary fibrosis can also be observed. RAB is not a P-glycoprotein substrate and does not penetrate the blood-brain barrier (VetDC Inc., personal communication).

SUMMARY

In summary, although companion animal lymphoma is a disease that can rarely be cured, it can be managed effectively in the majority of cases. Therapy is typically very well tolerated, and patients experience an excellent quality of life. Significant improvements have been made in recent years with regard to the treatment of this common disease, and we are hopeful that the coming years will bring equally great improvements.

CLINICS CARE POINTS

- CHOP-based chemotherapy remains the most efficacious first-line chemotherapy option for both dogs and cats with intermediate-grade to high-grade lymphoma.
- There is not a single rescue therapy option for canine lymphoma that integrates efficacy, cost, number of visits, and toxicity profile. In general, multi-agent protocols seem superior to single-agent treatment.
- The FDA-approved novel small molecules rabacfosadine (fully approved) and verdinexor (conditionally approved) are available in the United States for the treatment of canine lympmhoma. Studies are ongoing to optimize their use.

DISCLOSURE

Dr D.H. Thamm is a shareholder in and has received research funding from VetDC Inc., and is a paid consultant for Elanco, the developer and current distributor of rabacfosadine (Tanovea), respectively, which is discussed in this review.

REFERENCES

1. Rassnick KM, Bailey DB, Kamstock DA, et al. Survival time for dogs with previously untreated, peripheral nodal, intermediate- or large-cell lymphoma treated with prednisone alone: the Canine Lymphoma Steroid Only trial. J Am Vet Med Assoc 2021;259:62–71.
2. Lori JC, Stein TJ, Thamm DH. Doxorubicin and cyclophosphamide for the treatment of canine lymphoma: a randomized, placebo-controlled study. Vet Comp Oncol 2010;8:188–95.
3. Mutsaers AJ, Glickman NW, DeNicola DB, et al. Evaluation of treatment with doxorubicin and piroxicam or doxorubicin alone for multicentric lymphoma in dogs. J Am Vet Med Assoc 2002;220:1813–7.
4. Valerius KD, Ogilvie GK, Mallinckrodt CH, et al. Doxorubicin alone or in combination with asparaginase, followed by cyclophosphamide, vincristine, and prednisone for treatment of multicentric lymphoma in dogs: 121 cases (1987-1995). J Am Vet Med Assoc 1997;210:512–6.
5. Postorino NC, Susaneck SJ, Withrow SJ, et al. Single agent therapy with Adriamycin for canine lymphosarcoma. J Am Vet Med Assoc 1989;25:221–5.
6. Burton JH, Garrett-Mayer E, Thamm DH. Evaluation of a 15-week CHOP protocol for the treatment of canine multicentric lymphoma. Vet Comp Oncol 2013;11:306–15.
7. Curran K, Thamm DH. Retrospective analysis for treatment of naive canine multicentric lymphoma with a 15-week, maintenance-free CHOP protocol. Vet Comp Oncol 2016;14(Suppl 1):147–55.
8. Hosoya K, Kisseberth WC, Lord LK, et al. Comparison of COAP and UW-19 protocols for dogs with multicentric lymphoma. J Vet Intern Med 2007;21:1355–63.
9. MacDonald VS, Thamm DH, Kurzman ID, et al. Does L-asparaginase influence efficacy or toxicity when added to a standard CHOP protocol for dogs with lymphoma? J Vet Intern Med 2005;19:732–6.
10. Sorenmo K, Overley B, Krick E, et al. Outcome and toxicity associated with a dose-intensified, maintenance-free CHOP-based chemotherapy protocol in canine lymphoma: 130 cases. Vet Comp Oncol 2010;8:196–208.
11. Garrett LD, Thamm DH, Chun R, et al. Evaluation of a 6-month chemotherapy protocol with no maintenance therapy for dogs with lymphoma. J Vet Intern Med 2002;16:704–9.
12. Lautscham EM, Kessler M, Ernst T, et al. Comparison of a CHOP-LAsp-based protocol with and without maintenance for canine multicentric lymphoma. Vet Rec 2017;180:303.
13. Marconato L, Stefanello D, Valenti P, et al. Predictors of long-term survival in dogs with high-grade multicentric lymphoma. J Am Vet Med Assoc 2011;238:480–5.
14. Ruslander DA, Gebhard DH, Tompkins MB, et al. Immunophenotypic characterization of canine lymphoproliferative disorders. In Vivo 1997;11:169–72.
15. Teske E. Prognostic factors for malignant lymphoma in the dog: an update. Vet Q 1994;16(Suppl 1):29S–31S.
16. Sapierzynski R. Practical aspects of immunocytochemistry in canine lymphomas. Pol J Vet Sci 2010;13:661–8.
17. Rout ED, Avery PR. Lymphoid neoplasia: correlations between morphology and flow cytometry. Vet Clin North Am Small Anim Pract 2017;47:53–70.
18. Lana SE, Jackson TL, Burnett RC, et al. Utility of polymerase chain reaction for analysis of antigen receptor rearrangement in staging and predicting prognosis in dogs with lymphoma. J Vet Intern Med 2006;20:329–34.

19. Kristal O, Lana SE, Ogilvie GK, et al. Single agent chemotherapy with doxorubicin for feline lymphoma: a retrospective study of 19 cases (1994-1997). J Vet Intern Med 2001;15:125–30.

20. Peaston AE, Maddison JE. Efficacy of doxorubicin as an induction agent for cats with lymphosarcoma. Aust Vet J 1999;77:442–4.

21. Collette SA, Allstadt SD, Chon EM, et al. Treatment of feline intermediate- to high-grade lymphoma with a modified university of Wisconsin-Madison protocol: 119 cases (2004-2012). Vet Comp Oncol 2016;14(Suppl 1):136–46.

22. Limmer S, Eberle N, Nerschbach V, et al. Treatment of feline lymphoma using a 12-week, maintenance-free combination chemotherapy protocol in 26 cats. Vet Comp Oncol 2016;14(Suppl 1):21–31.

23. Kiselow MA, Rassnick KM, McDonough SP, et al. Outcome of cats with low-grade lymphocytic lymphoma: 41 cases (1995-2005). J Am Vet Med Assoc 2008;232: 405–10.

24. Pope KV, Tun AE, McNeill CJ, et al. Outcome and toxicity assessment of feline small cell lymphoma: 56 cases (2000-2010). Vet Med Sci 2015;1:51–62.

25. Stein TJ, Pellin M, Steinberg H, et al. Treatment of feline gastrointestinal small-cell lymphoma with chlorambucil and glucocorticoids. J Am Anim Hosp Assoc 2010; 46:413–7.

26. Flory AB, Rassnick KM, Erb HN, et al. Evaluation of factors associated with second remission in dogs with lymphoma undergoing retreatment with a cyclophosphamide, doxorubicin, vincristine, and prednisone chemotherapy protocol: 95 cases (2000-2007). J Am Vet Med Assoc 2011;238:501–6.

27. Lucroy MD, Phillips BS, Kraegel SA, et al. Evaluation of single-agent mitoxantrone as chemotherapy for relapsing canine lymphoma. J Vet Intern Med 1998;12: 325–9.

28. Moore AS, Ogilvie GK, Ruslander D, et al. Evaluation of mitoxantrone for the treatment of lymphoma in dogs. J Am Vet Med Assoc 1994;204:1903–5.

29. Ogilvie GK, Obradovich JE, Elmslie RE, et al. Efficacy of mitoxantrone against various neoplasms in dogs. J Am Vet Med Assoc 1991;198:1618–21.

30. Bannink EO, Sauerbrey ML, Mullins MN, et al. Actinomycin D as rescue therapy in dogs with relapsed or resistant lymphoma: 49 cases (1999–2006). J Am Vet Med Assoc 2008;233:446–51.

31. Moore AS, Ogilvie GK, Vail DM. Actinomycin D for reinduction of remission in dogs with resistant lymphoma. J Vet Intern Med 1994;8:343–4.

32. Moore AS, London CA, Wood CA, et al. Lomustine (CCNU) for the treatment of resistant lymphoma in dogs. J Vet Intern Med 1999;13:395–8.

33. Rusk A, Cozzi E, Stebbins M, et al. Cooperative activity of cytotoxic chemotherapy with antiangiogenic thrombospondin-I peptides, ABT-526 in pet dogs with relapsed lymphoma. Clin Cancer Res 2006;12:7456–64.

34. Griessmayr PC, Payne SE, Winter JE, et al. Dacarbazine as single-agent therapy for relapsed lymphoma in dogs. J Vet Intern Med 2009;23:1227–31.

35. Saba CF, Vickery KR, Clifford CA, et al. Rabacfosadine for relapsed canine B-cell lymphoma: Efficacy and adverse event profiles of 2 different doses. Vet Comp Oncol 2018;16:E76–82.

36. Vail DM, Thamm DH, Reiser H, et al. Assessment of GS-9219 in a pet dog model of non-Hodgkin's lymphoma. Clin Cancer Res 2009;15:3503–10.

37. Weishaar KM, Wright ZM, Rosenberg MP, et al. Multicenter, randomized, double-blinded, placebo-controlled study of rabacfosadine in dogs with lymphoma. J Vet Intern Med 2022;36:215–26.

38. Lenz JA, Robat CS, Stein TJ. Vinblastine as a second rescue for the treatment of canine multicentric lymphoma in 39 cases (2005 to 2014). J Small Anim Pract 2016;57:429–34.
39. Mastromauro ML, Suter SE, Hauck ML, et al. Oral melphalan for the treatment of relapsed canine lymphoma. Vet Comp Oncol 2018;16:E123–9.
40. Treggiari E, Elliott JW, Baines SJ, et al. Temozolomide alone or in combination with doxorubicin as a rescue agent in 37 cases of canine multicentric lymphoma. Vet Comp Oncol 2018;16:194–201.
41. Van Vechten M, Helfand SC, Jeglum KA. Treatment of relapsed canine lymphoma with doxorubicin and dacarbazine. J Vet Intern Med 1990;4:187–91.
42. Cawley JR, Wright ZM, Meleo K, et al. Concurrent use of rabacfosadine and L-asparaginase for relapsed or refractory multicentric lymphoma in dogs. J Vet Intern Med 2020;34:882–9.
43. Saba CF, Hafeman SD, Vail DM, et al. Combination chemotherapy with continuous L-asparaginase, lomustine, and prednisone for relapsed canine lymphoma. J Vet Intern Med 2009;23:1058–63.
44. Saba CF, Thamm DH, Vail DM. Combination chemotherapy with L-asparaginase, lomustine, and prednisone for relapsed or refractory canine lymphoma. J Vet Intern Med 2007;21:127–32.
45. Dervisis NG, Dominguez PA, Sarbu L, et al. Efficacy of temozolomide or dacarbazine in combination with an anthracycline for rescue chemotherapy in dogs with lymphoma. J Am Vet Med Assoc 2007;231:563–9.
46. Flory AB, Rassnick KM, Al-Sarraf R, et al. Combination of CCNU and DTIC chemotherapy for treatment of resistant lymphoma in dogs. J Vet Intern Med 2008;22:164–71.
47. Gillem J, Giuffrida M, Krick E. Efficacy and toxicity of carboplatin and cytarabine chemotherapy for dogs with relapsed or refractory lymphoma (2000-2013). Vet Comp Oncol 2017;15:400–10.
48. Batschinski K, Dervisis N, Kitchell B, et al. Combination of bleomycin and cytosine arabinoside chemotherapy for relapsed canine lymphoma. J Am Anim Hosp Assoc 2018;54:150–5.
49. Intile JL, Rassnick KM, Al-Sarraf R, et al. Evaluation of the tolerability of combination chemotherapy with mitoxantrone and dacarbazine in dogs with lymphoma. J Am Anim Hosp Assoc 2019;55:101–9.
50. O'Connell K, Thomson M, Morgan E, et al. Procarbazine, prednisolone and cyclophosphamide oral combination chemotherapy protocol for canine lymphoma. Vet Comp Oncol 2022;20:613–22.
51. Tanis JB, Mason SL, Maddox TW, et al. Evaluation of a multi-agent chemotherapy protocol combining lomustine, procarbazine and prednisolone (LPP) for the treatment of relapsed canine non-Hodgkin high-grade lymphomas. Vet Comp Oncol 2018;16:361–9.
52. Rassnick KM, Mauldin GE, Al-Sarraf R, et al. MOPP chemotherapy for treatment of resistant lymphoma in dogs: a retrospective study of 117 cases (1989-2000). J Vet Intern Med 2002;16:576–80.
53. Zimmerman K, Walsh KA, Ferrari JT, et al. Evaluation of mechlorethamine, vinblastine, procarbazine, and prednisone for the treatment of resistant multicentric canine lymphoma. Vet Comp Oncol 2023;21(3):503–8.
54. Smallwood K, Tanis JB, Grant IA, et al. Evaluation of a multi-agent chemotherapy protocol combining dexamethasone, melphalan, actinomycin D, and cytarabine for the treatment of resistant canine non-Hodgkin high-grade lymphomas: a single centre's experience. Vet Comp Oncol 2019;17:165–73.

55. Alvarez FJ, Kisseberth WC, Gallant SL, et al. Dexamethasone, melphalan, actinomycin D, cytosine arabinoside (DMAC) protocol for dogs with relapsed lymphoma. J Vet Intern Med 2006;20:1178–83.

56. Parsons-Doherty M, Poirier VJ, Monteith G. The efficacy and adverse event profile of dexamethasone, melphalan, actinomycin D, and cytosine arabinoside (DMAC) chemotherapy in relapsed canine lymphoma. Can Vet J 2014;55:175–80.

57. LeBlanc AK, Mauldin GE, Milner RJ, et al. Efficacy and toxicity of BOPP and LOPP chemotherapy for the treatment of relapsed canine lymphoma. Vet Comp Oncol 2006;4:21–32.

58. Fahey CE, Milner RJ, Barabas K, et al. Evaluation of the University of Florida lomustine, vincristine, procarbazine, and prednisone chemotherapy protocol for the treatment of relapsed lymphoma in dogs: 33 cases (2003-2009). J Am Vet Med Assoc 2011;239:209–15.

59. Back AR, Schleis SE, Smrkovski OA, et al. Mechlorethamine, vincristine, melphalan and prednisone (MOMP) for the treatment of relapsed lymphoma in dogs. Vet Comp Oncol 2015;13:398–408.

60. Kim C, Wouda RM, Borrego J, et al. Cyclophosphamide rescue therapy for relapsed low-grade alimentary lymphoma after chlorambucil treatment in cats. J Feline Med Surg 2021;23:976–86.

61. Smallwood K, Harper A, Blackwood L. Lomustine, methotrexate and cytarabine chemotherapy as a rescue treatment for feline lymphoma. J Feline Med Surg 2021;23:722–9.

62. Elliott J, Finotello R. A dexamethasone, melphalan, actinomycin-D and cytarabine chemotherapy protocol as a rescue treatment for feline lymphoma. Vet Comp Oncol 2018;16:E144–51.

63. Martin OA, Price J. Mechlorethamine, vincristine, melphalan and prednisolone rescue chemotherapy protocol for resistant feline lymphoma. J Feline Med Surg 2018;20:934–9.

64. Dutelle AL, Bulman-Fleming JC, Lewis CA, et al. Evaluation of lomustine as a rescue agent for cats with resistant lymphoma. J Feline Med Surg 2012;14:694–700.

65. Jeffreys AB, Knapp DW, Carlton WW, et al. Influence of asparaginase on a combination chemotherapy protocol for canine multicentric lymphoma. J Am Anim Hosp Assoc 2005;41:221–6.

66. Warry E, Hansen RJ, Gustafson DL, et al. Pharmacokinetics of cyclophosphamide after oral and intravenous administration to dogs with lymphoma. J Vet Intern Med 2011;25:903–8.

67. Stroda KA, Murphy JD, Hansen RJ, et al. Pharmacokinetics of cyclophosphamide and 4-hydroxycyclophosphamide in cats after oral, intravenous, and intraperitoneal administration of cyclophosphamide. Am J Vet Res 2017;78:862–6.

68. Childress MO, Ramos-Vara JA, Ruple A. A randomized controlled trial of the effect of prednisone omission from a multidrug chemotherapy protocol on treatment outcome in dogs with peripheral nodal lymphomas. J Am Vet Med Assoc 2016;249:1067–78.

69. Zandvliet M, Rutteman GR, Teske E. Prednisolone inclusion in a first-line multidrug cytostatic protocol for the treatment of canine lymphoma does not affect therapy results. Vet J 2013;197:656–61.

70. Risbon RE, de Lorimier LP, Skorupski K, et al. Response of canine cutaneous epitheliotropic lymphoma to lomustine (CCNU): a retrospective study of 46 cases (1999-2004). J Vet Intern Med 2006;20:1389–97.

71. Williams LE, Rassnick KM, Power HT, et al. CCNU in the treatment of canine epitheliotropic lymphoma. J Vet Intern Med 2006;20:136–43.
72. Flood-Knapik KE, Durham AC, Gregor TP, et al. Clinical, histopathological and immunohistochemical characterization of canine indolent lymphoma. Vet Comp Oncol 2013;11:272–86.
73. Lane J, Price J, Moore A, et al. Low-grade gastrointestinal lymphoma in dogs: 20 cases (2010 to 2016). J Small Anim Pract 2018;59:147–53.
74. Sauerbrey ML, Mullins MN, Bannink EO, et al. Lomustine and prednisone as a first-line treatment for dogs with multicentric lymphoma: 17 cases (2004-2005). J Am Vet Med Assoc 2007;230:1866–9.
75. Beaver LM, Strottner G, Klein MK. Response rate after administration of a single dose of doxorubicin in dogs with B-cell or T-cell lymphoma: 41 cases (2006-2008). J Am Vet Med Assoc 2010;237:1052–5.
76. Brown PM, Tzannes S, Nguyen S, et al. LOPP chemotherapy as a first-line treatment for dogs with T-cell lymphoma. Vet Comp Oncol 2018;16:108–13.
77. Morgan E, O'Connell K, Thomson M, Griffin A. Canine T cell lymphoma treated with lomustine, vincristine, procarbazine, and prednisolone chemotherapy in 35 dogs. Vet Comp Oncol 2018;16(4):622–9.
78. Brodsky EM, Maudlin GN, Lachowicz JL, et al. Asparaginase and MOPP treatment of dogs with lymphoma. J Vet Intern Med 2009;23:578–84.
79. Rebhun RB, Kent MS, Borrofka SA, et al. CHOP chemotherapy for the treatment of canine multicentric T-cell lymphoma. Vet Comp Oncol 2011;9:38–44.
80. Krick EL, Cohen RB, Gregor TP, et al. Prospective clinical trial to compare vincristine and vinblastine in a COP-based protocol for lymphoma in cats. J Vet Intern Med 2013;27:134–40.
81. Mahony OM, Moore AS, Cotter SM, et al. Alimentary lymphoma in cats: 28 cases (1988-1993). J Am Vet Med Assoc 1995;207:1593–8.
82. Waite AH, Jackson K, Gregor TP, et al. Lymphoma in cats treated with a weekly cyclophosphamide-, vincristine-, and prednisone-based protocol: 114 cases (1998-2008). J Am Vet Med Assoc 2013;242:1104–9.
83. Rau SE, Burgess KE. A retrospective evaluation of lomustine (CeeNU) in 32 treatment naive cats with intermediate to large cell gastrointestinal lymphoma (2006-2013). Vet Comp Oncol 2017;15:1019–28.
84. Frimberger AE, Moore AS, Rassnick KM, et al. A combination chemotherapy protocol with dose intensification and autologous bone marrow transplant (VELCAP-HDC) for canine lymphoma. J Vet Intern Med 2006;20:355–64.
85. Warry EE, Willcox JL, Suter SE. Autologous peripheral blood hematopoietic cell transplantation in dogs with T-cell lymphoma. J Vet Intern Med 2014;28:529–37.
86. Willcox JL, Pruitt A, Suter SE. Autologous peripheral blood hematopoietic cell transplantation in dogs with B-cell lymphoma. J Vet Intern Med 2012;26:1155–63.
87. Gareau A, Sekiguchi T, Warry E, et al. Allogeneic peripheral blood haematopoietic stem cell transplantation for the treatment of dogs with high-grade B-cell lymphoma. Vet Comp Oncol 2022;20:862–70.
88. Coiffier B, Lepage E, Briere J, et al. CHOP chemotherapy plus rituximab compared with CHOP alone in elderly patients with diffuse large-B-cell lymphoma. N Engl J Med 2002;346:235–42.
89. Pfreundschuh M, Trumper L, Osterborg A, et al. CHOP-like chemotherapy plus rituximab versus CHOP-like chemotherapy alone in young patients with good-prognosis diffuse large-B-cell lymphoma: a randomised controlled trial by the MabThera International Trial (MInT) Group. Lancet Oncol 2006;7:379–91.

90. Lim SH, Levy R. Translational medicine in action: anti-CD20 therapy in lymphoma. J Immunol 2014;193:1519–24.

91. Rue SM, Eckelman BP, Efe JA, et al. Identification of a candidate therapeutic antibody for treatment of canine B-cell lymphoma. Vet Immunol Immunopathol 2015; 164:148–59.

92. Weiskopf K, Anderson KL, Ito D, et al. Eradication of canine diffuse large B-cell lymphoma in a murine xenograft model with CD47 blockade and anti-CD20. Cancer Immunol Res 2016;4:1072–87.

93. Sadowski AR, Gardner HL, Borgatti A, et al. Phase II study of the oral selective inhibitor of nuclear export (SINE) KPT-335 (verdinexor) in dogs with lymphoma. BMC Vet Res 2018;14:250.

94. Reiser H, Wang J, Chong L, et al. GS-9219–a novel acyclic nucleotide analogue with potent antineoplastic activity in dogs with spontaneous non-Hodgkin's lymphoma. Clin Cancer Res 2008;14:2824–32.

95. Thamm DH, Vail DM, Post GS, et al. Alternating rabacfosadine/doxorubicin: efficacy and tolerability in naive canine multicentric lymphoma. J Vet Intern Med 2017;31:872–8.

96. Morges MA, Burton JH, Saba CF, et al. Phase II evaluation of VDC-1101 in canine cutaneous T-cell lymphoma. J Vet Intern Med 2014;28:1569–74.

Veterinary Interventional Oncology

William T.N. Culp, VMD

KEYWORDS

- Interventional radiology • Neoplasia • Embolization • Stenting

KEY POINTS

- Interventional radiology (IR) is a specialty focused on using image-guidance to direct the performance of procedures in companion animals.
- Interventional oncology is a subspecialty of IR focused on diagnosis and treatment of neoplastic disease.
- Locoregional therapies such as directed vascular therapy and ablation can be used for the treatment of multiple neoplastic conditions in companion animals and provide a less-invasive alternative to surgery.
- Stenting of malignant obstructions is commonly performed in companion animals and seems to be both highly tolerated and effective.

OVERVIEW

The use of traditional cancer therapies such as surgery, chemotherapy, and radiation therapy are well established in veterinary medicine. Although more recently accepted for cancer diagnosis and treatment, interventional oncology (IO) techniques have now established a foothold as well and are often part of the conversations that veterinarians have with colleagues and companion animal caretakers about their pets with cancer. Options such as stenting of malignant obstructions have now been used in veterinary medicine for approximately a quarter century. Locoregional therapies such as intra-arterial chemotherapy delivery, embolization, and ablation are more recently developing options but early results are highly promising.

Anatomy

A thorough knowledge of the anatomy is essential for performing IO procedures effectively and safely. Introduction of instrumentation into and navigation through luminal structures requires an excellent understanding of anatomic landmarks and organ interaction. Additionally, the blood supply to various organs should be understood

University of California-Davis, School of Veterinary Medicine, One Garrod Drive, Davis, CA 95616, USA
E-mail address: wculp@ucdavis.edu

Vet Clin Small Anim 54 (2024) 491–500
https://doi.org/10.1016/j.cvsm.2023.12.005
0195-5616/24/© 2023 Elsevier Inc. All rights reserved.
vetsmall.theclinics.com

when transcatheter locoregional therapies are being considered so that normal blood supply can be identified from tumoral blood supply and complications such as nontarget embolization can be avoided. The arterial blood supply of the abdominal organs has been fluoroscopically described as a guide for performing intra-abdominal transcatheter therapies.[1]

Currently, access for the majority of vascular-based locoregional therapies in veterinary patients is from the arteries (eg, carotid and femoral arteries). If vascular stenting is being performed, the jugular or femoral vein may also be used. Venous approaches do not require vascular repair postprocedure due to the low pressure in the venous system; however, arterial approaches generally require vessel ligation or repair. In humans, closure of an arteriotomy site is often performed with a vascular closure device; vascular closure devices are generally not used in veterinary patients due to expense, the need for minimized postprocedure patient activity, and the fact that the femoral and carotid arteries can be ligated.[2–4]

Imaging diagnostics

The use of imaging modalities to guide IO procedures allows for procedures to be performed in a minimally invasive fashion and improves a clinician's ability to access certain organs or regions of the body. Fluoroscopy is used during the majority of IO procedures in companion animals. The instrumentation used during IO procedures is radiopaque and contrast agents are often injected intraluminally or intravascularly making fluoroscopy an excellent modality for performing real-time interventions.

Ultrasonography is regularly used as a means of cancer staging, specifically in the abdomen; further, ultrasound guidance can provide crucial assistance in obtaining tissue samples via fine-needle aspiration or biopsy. Ultrasound can also be used to locate blood vessels for percutaneous vascular catheterization and is the most likely imaging modality to be used to perform percutaneous tumor ablation.[5] Additionally, for percutaneous ureteral stenting, ultrasound is used to guide percutaneous access into the renal pelvis.[6]

Similar to ultrasound, computed tomography (CT) and MRI are essential components of patient staging and preprocedural planning in veterinary medicine. These advanced imaging modalities are often combined with fluoroscopic imaging in human medicine to allow for real-time evaluation and treatment of lesions. Computed tomography angiography and magnetic resonance angiography are used in the evaluation of veterinary patients regularly but intraprocedural use of these diagnostics remains less common.

PATIENT SELECTION

When possible and appropriate, IO techniques should be considered in addition to more traditional options such as surgery, chemotherapy, and radiation therapy. Because most patients diagnosed with cancer are older, procedures that cause the least amount of morbidity are ideal. In many scenarios in which IO options are offered, these techniques are the only available option. IO procedures have the benefit of often being performed in a minimally invasive fashion; the overall goal is to improve quality of life after recovery when one of these techniques is selected.

PROCEDURES

The areas of IO that have received the majority of attention thus far in veterinary medicine include locoregional therapies (intra-arterial chemotherapy, embolization/chemoembolization, and ablative therapies) and stenting of malignant obstructions.

Other palliative treatments such as the draining of malignant effusions and normal fluid accumulations have also been performed.

LOCOREGIONAL THERAPIES
Intra-arterial Chemotherapy

The administration of chemotherapy in veterinary patients is generally performed intra-venously. However, the intra-arterial delivery of chemotherapy can provide some theoretic advantages over traditional administration. When a drug is delivered intra-arterially, the tumor receives a maximized dose thus allowing for a higher concentration to accumulate in the tumor.[7–9] Additionally, drugs that are administered intrave-nously have been shown to have higher systemic concentrations and side effects of chemotherapy may occur more commonly.[7–9] Despite the proposed advantages, intra-arterial chemotherapy is still not universally used in human medicine, although some locations, particularly the head and neck region, have shown promise.

To perform the procedure, a sheath is placed within the artery that has been chosen. Using varying sizes and types of guidewires and catheters, the vascular supply of the affected organ is accessed via superselective catheterization. Once the desired vessel is selected, chemotherapy can be administered (**Fig. 1**) increasing the locally delivered dose.

Although still uncommonly used in companion animals, a study has compared the response to intra-arterial or intravenous administration of chemotherapy in the treatment of lower urinary tract neoplasia in dogs.[10] In the dogs of that study, there was a significantly greater decrease in tumor size in the dogs of the intra-arterial chemotherapy group as compared with the intravenous chemotherapy group. Additionally, dogs in the intra-arterial group were less likely to develop side effects such as anemia, lethargy, and anorexia.[10] However, this study only evaluated the short-term response to these therapies and used ultrasound, which has demonstrated previous limitations, as the imaging modality for measurement.

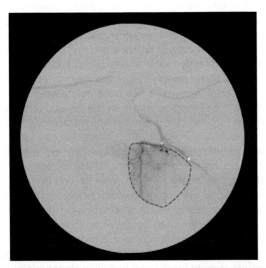

Fig. 1. Lateral fluoroscopic image acquired during an intra-arterial chemotherapy treatment in a 10-year-old male castrated pit bull terrier with urothelial carcinoma of the prostate (*red dashed line*), urethra, and bladder trigone. The catheter has been placed in a location where chemotherapy can be delivered to both the prostatic arterial branches (+) and the caudal vesical artery (*asterisk*), which is supplying blood to the bladder.

Another use of intra-arterial chemotherapy in human patients is in combination with radiation therapy.[11] Drugs such as platinum-based chemotherapy agents can "sensitize" tumors to the effects of radiation therapy, and the goal of combining therapies is to maximize the efficacy. In veterinary patients, the use of radiation therapy in combination with intra-arterial chemotherapy has been evaluated in both patients with osteosarcoma and patients with bladder cancer.[12–15] In one of the appendicular osteosarcoma studies, the toxicity associated with chemotherapy administration and radiation side effects were rare, and median survival time in these dogs was 9.3 months.[15] Dogs with greater than 75% tumor necrosis had significantly lower recurrence rates at 1 year (15%) versus dogs with less than 75% tumor necrosis (65%).[15] In a separate study comparing different treatments for canine osteosarcoma including intra-arterial chemotherapy alone and intra-arterial chemotherapy with radiation therapy, the percent of tumor necrosis was 49.1% and 83.7%, respectively, for those treatment categories.[14] Another study documented a median survival time of 6.7 months in dogs receiving intra-arterial cisplatin chemotherapy in conjunction with radiation therapy as an alternative to amputation or limb-sparing surgery.[12] In a study evaluating the combination of intra-arterial chemotherapy (cisplatin) with radiation therapy for the treatment of bladder cancer, 2 dogs demonstrated an objective reduction in tumor size.[13] Side effects and toxicity were minimal in these 2 dogs.[13]

Embolization/Chemoembolization

Embolotherapy is an established treatment modality in human oncology and is considered a standard-of-care therapy for some tumors. The reasoning behind embolization is that localized, tumor-specific ischemia will lead to tumor cell death. The addition of chemotherapy to embolization (ie, chemoembolization) theoretically further increases tumor cell death due to the cytotoxic properties of chemotherapy.

Embolization performed without chemotherapy is often referred to as transarterial embolization (TAE) or "bland" embolization. When transarterial chemoembolization (TACE) is preformed, chemotherapy can be delivered in conjunction with the embolic agent (conventional TACE) or delivered via beads (drug-eluting bead TACE or DEB-TACE) that have been loaded with chemotherapy (eg, doxorubicin). Radioembolization is a developing embolotherapy in humans and involves the delivery of radioactive particles (eg, Yttrium-90) directly to the arterial blood supply of a tumor.[16]

The liver has a unique blood supply in that the majority of the blood supplying the liver comes from the portal vein, yet it has been established that tumors in the liver receive the majority of their blood supply from the hepatic arteries.[17] This allows for targeting of the major tumoral blood supply while preserving blood flow to normal tissue.

To perform liver embolization/chemoembolization, the arterial blood supply is accessed from the femoral or carotid artery. Using fluoroscopy and serial angiographic studies, the hepatic artery (second order branch from the aorta) is selected, and an angiographic map of the hepatic tumoral blood supply is obtained. Once the hepatic arterial branch (or branches) that is supplying the tumor is identified, the embolic agent (± chemotherapy) can be delivered to the tumor.

In companion animals, embolization of liver tumors has been the most commonly reported embolization technique to date.[18–23] In the earliest 2 studies, several mixtures of chemoembolic agents were used including doxorubicin/iodized oil, doxorubicin/mitomycin/iodized oil/polyvinyl alcohol particles, doxorubicin/iodized oil/polyvinyl alcohol particles, and polyvinyl alcohol particles alone.[18,19] Survival times postprocedure were available in 3 out of 4 dogs and ranged from 28 to 137 days. Stable disease or subjective decreases in tumor size were noted in several of the cases.[18,19] In a study of dogs undergoing bland embolization, median survival time (MST) after embolization was 419 days and a history of intra-abdominal hemorrhage and pre-TAE tumor volume/body weight were significantly associated with survival.[23] In 2 studies evaluating DEB-TACE with either doxorubicin or paclitaxel, MSTs have varied between 337 days[20] and 629 days,[22] respectively. Postembolization tumor volume reduction after TAE/DEB-TACE has been reported in the 13% to 51% range but follow-up time has varied.[20,22,23]

Prostatic artery embolization (PAE) has been established as a viable and effective treatment option for prostate neoplasia during the last several years. To perform PAE, the prostatic arterial blood supply is selected bilaterally with the aim of causing permanent cessation of blood flow to the prostate (**Fig. 2**). The overall goal is to improve clinical signs and control local disease in the long term. Recently, a prospective study evaluated 20 dogs undergoing PAE.[24] All dogs demonstrated a decrease in prostatic volume as measured with CT, and significant improvement in multiple clinical signs was noted. No major complications were encountered.[24]

Although treatment of nasal tumors with radiation therapy is considered by most as the treatment of choice, embolization can also be considered and is often pursued at the author's clinic. As the blood supply to the nasal cavity can be isolated, embolization tends to be highly tolerated.

Ablation

Descriptions of the use of tumor ablation have been sparse in the veterinary literature but the proven applications in human patients open the door for possible uses in animals as well. Ablative techniques function via chemical or thermal destruction of tumor cells. Chemical ablation techniques generally involve the intratumoral injection of liquid agents, with ethanol being the most described technique. Thermal ablation is based on the delivery of energy or freezing agents directly to a tumor to incite cell death.

The major thermal ablative techniques that are used include radiofrequency ablation (RFA), cryoablation, microwave ablation (MWA), laser ablation and high-intensity

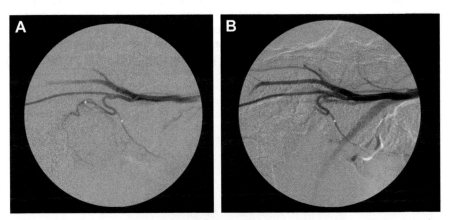

Fig. 2. Lateral fluoroscopic images of a 13-year-old male castrated Belgian Malinois undergoing PAE. (*A*) Preembolization: The prostatic arterial blood supply (+) and caudal vesical artery (*asterisk*) can be visualized before embolization. (*B*) Postembolization: After embolization of the prostatic arterial blood supply only the blood supply to the bladder (*asterisk*) can be visualized.

focused ultrasound. With the above techniques that generate heat, tumor death is caused by the transfer of heat to tumor cells with subsequent necrosis.[25] When performing cryoablation, varying freeze–thaw cycles result in the development of intracellular ice crystals and cellular dehydration, both of which lead to cellular damage and death.[25]

With RFA, cryoablation, and MWA, probes are often introduced into tumor tissue percutaneously (**Fig. 3**) or through a natural orifice. Guidance of the probes into the appropriate location is performed with image-guidance, which may include fluoroscopy, CT or MRI, although ultrasound is generally the most used imaging modality. These procedures can also be performed with direct access to the tumor, for example, after a celiotomy or with endoscopic-guidance.

RFA and cryoablation are commonly used in human patients in the treatment of hepatic, prostate, kidney, and bone tumors, among many others.[26,27] However, descriptions of the use of these modalities in the treatment of companion animal malignancies beyond case reports are rare. In the author's clinic, a metastatic carcinoma lesion to the prostate was treated successfully via RFA, and there have been 2 reported cases of cryoablation in the treatment of nasal and maxillary tumors.[28,29] In a report of the use of cryoablation to treat a recurrent nasal adenocarcinoma, long-term tumor control was achieved.[28] In that case, probe placement was guided with fluoroscopy and CT, and tumor response was monitored by CT. Clinical signs were mild and included epiphora in the periprocedural period and mild chronic nasal discharge.[28] Combination therapy with TAE, systemic cyclophosphamide, and cryoablation was used to treat a dog with a maxillary fibrosarcoma; partial tumor remission was noted at a 4-week recheck examination.[29]

MWA holds tremendous potential for use in companion animals and several advantages over other modalities such as RFA have been noted including the ability to generate higher intratumoral temperatures, faster ablations, less char and potentially less pain; additionally, as opposed to RFA, MWA does not require pads to be placed on the skin, which can be challenging in smaller patients. The use of MWA in companion animals has been combined with open and laparoscopic/thoracoscopic surgeries[30–32] as well as percutaneously.[5,33] In 7 dogs with liver neoplasia undergoing MWA, complications were not reported and overall response was encouraging.[30,32] Three dogs with retroperitoneal masses were successfully treated with percutaneous MWA and no major complications were encountered.[5] Local recurrence was not noted in any dog. In a dog with metastatic pulmonary disease and secondary hypertrophic osteopathy, resolution of the clinical signs associated with hypertrophic osteopathy was noted post-MWA.[31]

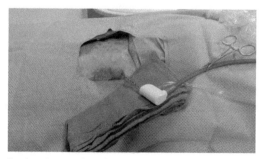

Fig. 3. A MWA probe has been placed percutaneously with ultrasound-guidance into a retroperitoneal mass of a 11-year-old female spayed mixed breed dog.

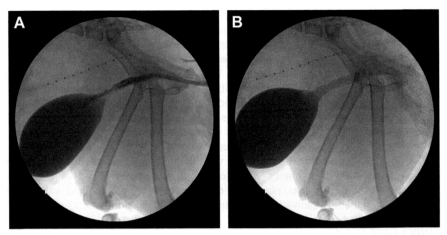

Fig. 4. Urethral stent placement in an 11-year-old female pit bull terrier. (*A*) A contrast cystourethrogram has been performed, and a stricture in the region of the trigone and proximal urethra secondary to a urothelial carcinoma can be seen. (*B*) After stent placement, luminal patency has been reestablished.

STENTING OF MALIGNANT OBSTRUCTIONS

A stent is a tube-like device that recanalizes a luminal obstruction. Stents reestablish an opening to allow for the excretion of body fluids or waste, as well as for the passage of food, liquid, air, or blood. Stents have provided a highly effective treatment option for opening malignant obstructions in companion animals. Additionally, stents can be placed intraluminally in minimally invasive fashion and recovery is generally rapid.

Urethral stenting is likely one of the most common applications of IO in veterinary medicine (**Fig. 4**). The importance of urethral stenting lies in the ability of the stent to palliate a condition that is immediately life-threatening, specifically uretheral obstruction with resultant urine retention. With many cases of urinary tract obstruction secondary to neoplasia (tumors of the prostate, bladder, and urethra), the cause of death is the severity of local disease as opposed to metastasis.

Several clinical studies have described the use of urethral stents in canine and feline patients.[34–37] These studies found that urethral stents can successfully be placed through a natural orifice in canine patients with lower urinary tract neoplasia and can effectively reestablish urine flow. The most common complication encountered in dogs is incontinence. In female cats and male cats with a previous perineal urethrostomy, placement of urethral stents can be performed in a retrograde manner through the urethral opening. In unaltered male cats, a small cystotomy is likely necessary as the instrumentation is too large to fit through the typical penile urethral orifice.

Ureteral stenting of malignant obstruction in dogs is generally pursued when a lower urinary tract neoplasia (bladder, urethra, or prostate tumor) has grown into a position where the ureteral orifice is unilaterally or bilaterally covered resulting in obstruction with secondary hydroureter and/or hydronephrosis. A percutaneous antegrade approach for the placement of ureteral stents has been described.[6] In one study evaluating outcomes in 12 dogs with ureteral obstruction, results were promising in that stents were able to be placed in all dogs and complications were rare; additionally, all dogs were discharged and in those that had follow-up ultrasound, hydronephrosis, and hydroureter were improved in all.[6] In the author's experience, ureteral stents placed for the treatment of malignant obstructions in cats are most effectively placed after a celiotomy; guide wire placement across the obstruction (before stent passage) is still most easily performed via an antegrade approach despite a celiotomy being performed.

Surgical resection of colonic, esophageal, and tracheal tumors is the treatment of choice for tumors affecting these organs. With extensive luminal obstruction or large tumor burden, removal is not always possible, and stenting can be considered to allow for patency. Vascular stents can be placed to palliate obstructions from large tumors or complications associated with previous surgeries. Vascular obstruction of veins is more likely to occur, and descriptions of vascular stenting in veterinary cases have mostly focused on hepatic vein and vena cava obstruction.[38,39] In one case series of 3 dogs with Budd-Chiari syndrome, vascular patency was reestablished after image-guided stent placement.[38] Additionally, in a dog diagnosed with a heart-based tumor and chylothorax, placement of a transatrial stent combined with stereotactic radiation therapy allowed for resolution of chylothorax and prolonged survival.[39]

CLINICS CARE POINT

- When considering therapies for diseases that seem to lack traditional treatment options, consulting with someone who has experience with Interventional Oncology may yield further strategies to pursue.

DISCLOSURE

The author declares no commercial or financial conflicts of interest, and no funding was received for this study.

REFERENCES

1. Culp WTN, Mayhew PD, Pascoe PJ, et al. Angiographic anatomy of the major abdominal arterial blood supply in the dog. Vet Radiol Ultrasound 2015;56: 474–85.
2. Clendenin MA, Conrad MC. Collateral vessel development, following unilateral chronic carotid occlusion in the dog. Am J Vet Res 1979;40:84–8.
3. Clendenin MA, Conrad MC. Collateral vessel development after chronic bilateral common carotid artery occlusion in the dog. Am J Vet Res 1979;40:1244–8.
4. Perkins RL, Edmark KW. Ligation of femoral vessels and azygous vein in the dog. J Am Vet Med Assoc 1971;159:993–4.
5. Culp WTN, Johnson EG, Palm CA, et al. Use of percutaneous microwave ablation in the treatment of retroperitoneal neoplasia in three dogs. J Am Vet Med Assoc 2021;259:1171–7.
6. Berent AC, Weisse C, Beal MW, et al. Use of indwelling, double-pigtail stents for treatment of malignant ureteral obstruction in dogs: 12 cases (2006-2009). J Am Vet Med Assoc 2011;238:1017–25.
7. Chen C, Wang W, Zhou H, et al. Pharmacokinetic comparison between systemic and local chemotherapy by carboplatin in dogs. Reprod Sci 2009;16:1097–102.
8. von Scheel J, Golde G. Pharmacokinetics of intra-arterial tumour therapy. An experimental study. Arch Oto-Rhino-Laryngol 1984;239:153–61.
9. von Scheel J, Krautzberger W, Foth B, et al. A special method of intra-arterial infusion for treatment of head and neck cancer. Recent Results Cancer Res 1983;86: 169–73.

10. Culp WT, Weisse C, Berent AC, et al. Early tumor response to intraarterial or intravenous administration of carboplatin to treat naturally occurring lower urinary tract carcinoma in dogs. J Vet Intern Med 2015;29:900–7.

11. Samant S, Robbins KT, Vang M, et al. Intra-arterial cisplatin and concomitant radiation therapy followed by surgery for advanced paranasal sinus cancer. Arch Otolaryngol Head Neck Surg 2004;130:948–55.

12. Heidner GL, Page RL, McEntee MC, et al. Treatment of canine appendicular osteosarcoma using cobalt 60 radiation and intraarterial cisplatin. J Vet Intern Med 1991;5:313–6.

13. McCaw DL, Lattimer JC. Radiation and cisplatin for treatment of canine urinary bladder carcinoma. Vet Radiol 1988;29:264–8.

14. Powers BE, Withrow SJ, Thrall DE, et al. Percent tumor necrosis as a predictor of treatment response in canine osteosarcoma. Cancer 1991;67:126–34.

15. Withrow SJ, Thrall DE, Straw RC, et al. Intra-arterial cisplatin with or without radiation in limb-sparing for canine osteosarcoma. Cancer 1993;71:2484–90.

16. Aliseda D, Marti-Cruchaga P, Zozaya G, et al. Liver resection and transplantation following Yttrium-90 radioembolization for primary malignant liver tumors: a 15-year single-center experience. Cancers 2023;15. https://doi.org/10.3390/cancers15030733.

17. Breedis C, Young G. The blood supply of neoplasms in the liver. Am J Pathol 1954;30:969–85.

18. Weisse C, Clifford C, Holt D, et al. Percutaneous arterial embolization and chemoembolization for treatment of benign and malignant tumors in three dogs and a goat. J Am Vet Med Assoc 2002;221:1430–6.

19. Cave TA, Johnson V, Beths T, et al. Treatment of unresectable hepatocellular adenoma in dogs with transarterial iodized oil and chemotherapy with and without an embolic agent: a report of two cases. Vet Comp Oncol 2003;1:191–9.

20. Rogatko CP, Weisse C, Schwarz T, et al. Drug-eluting bead chemoembolization for the treatment of nonresectable hepatic carcinoma in dogs: a prospective clinical trial. J Vet Intern Med 2021;35:1487–95.

21. Samuel N, Weisse C, Berent AC, et al. Pharmacokinetic study comparing doxorubicin concentrations after chemoembolization or intravenous administration in dogs with naturally occurring nonresectable hepatic carcinoma. J Vet Intern Med 2022;36:1792–9.

22. Culp WTN, Johnson EG, Giuffrida MA, et al. Evaluation of the use of a novel bioabsorbable polymer drug-eluting microsphere for transarterial embolization of hepatocellular neoplasia in dogs. PLoS One 2022;17:e0269941.

23. Kawamura Y, Itou H, Kida A, et al. Therapeutic response and prognostic factors of 14 dogs undergoing transcatheter arterial embolization for hepatocellular masses: a retrospective study. J Vet Intern Med 2023;37:1455–65.

24. Culp WTN, Johnson EG, Giuffrida MA, et al. Procedural description and prospective evalaution of short-term outcome for the use of prostatic artery embolization in dogs with carcinoma of the prostate. J Am Vet Med Assoc 2021;259:1154–62.

25. Bhardwaj N, Strickland AD, Ahmad F, et al. Liver ablation techniques: a review. Surg Endosc 2010;24:254–65.

26. Nazario J, Hernandez J, Tam AL. Thermal ablation of painful bone metastases. Tech Vasc Interv Radiol 2011;14:150–9.

27. Callstrom MR, Kurup AN. Percutaneous ablation for bone and soft tissue metastases-why cryoablation? Skeletal Radiol 2009;38:835–9.

28. Murphy SM, Lawrence JA, Schmiedt CW, et al. Image-guided transnasal cryoablation of a recurrent nasal adenocarcinoma in a dog. J Small Anim Pract 2011; 52:329–33.

29. Weisse C, Solomon S. Combined transarterial embolization, systemic cyclophosphamide, and cryotherapy ablation for "Hi-Lo" maxillary fibrosarcoma in a dog. San Pedro, Belize: Proceedings: 8th Annual Meeting, Veterinary Endoscopy Society; May 5-7, 2011.

30. Yang Y, Wang C, Lu Y, et al. Outcomes of ultrasound-guided percutaneous argon-helium cryoablation of hepatocellular carcinoma. J Hepato-Biliary-Pancreatic Sci 2012;19:674–84.

31. Mazzaccari K, Boston SE, Toskich BB, et al. Video-assisted microwave ablation for the treatment of a metastatic lung lesion in a dog with appendicular osteosarcoma and hypertrophic osteopathy. Vet Surg 2017;46:1161–5.

32. Oramas A, Case JB, Toskich BB, et al. Laparoscopic access to the liver and application of laparoscopic microwave ablation in 2 dogs with liver neoplasia. Vet Surg 2019;48:O91–8.

33. Dornbusch JA, Wavreille VA, Dent B, et al. Percutaneous microwave ablation of solitary presumptive pulmonary metastases in two dogs with appendicular osteosarcoma. Vet Surg 2020;49:1174–82.

34. Weisse C, Berent A, Todd K, et al. Evaluation of palliative stenting for management of malignant urethral obstructions in dogs. J Am Vet Med Assoc 2006; 229:226–34.

35. McMillan SK, Knapp DW, Ramos-Vara JA, et al. Outcome of urethral stent placement for management of urethral obstruction secondary to transitional cell carcinoma in dogs: 19 cases (2007-2010). J Am Vet Med Assoc 2012;241:1627–32.

36. Blackburn AL, Berent AC, Weisse CW, et al. Evaluation of outcome following urethral stent placement for the treatment of obstructive carcinoma of the urethra in dogs: 42 cases (2004-2008). J Am Vet Med Assoc 2013;242:59–68.

37. Brace MA, Weisse C, Berent A. Preliminary experience with stenting for management of non-urolith urethral obstruction in eight cats. Vet Surg 2014;43:199–208.

38. Schlicksup MD, Weisse CW, Berent AC, et al. Use of endovascular stents in three dogs with Budd-Chiari syndrome. J Am Vet Med Assoc 2009;235:544–50.

39. Gibson EA, Culp WTN, Kent MS, et al. Treatment of a heart base tumor and chylothorax with endovascular stent, stereotactic body radiation therapy, and a tyrosine kinase inhibitor in a dog. J Vet Cardiol 2021;33:61–8.

Precision Medicine in Veterinary Science

Esther Chon, DVM[a], William Hendricks, PhD[a],
Michelle White, DVM, PhD[b], Lucas Rodrigues, DVM, PhD[b],
David Haworth, DVM, PhD[a], Gerald Post, DVM, MEM[b],*

KEYWORDS

- Targeted therapy • Genomics • Personalized medicine • Individualized medicine
- Genomic panels • Dogs • Canine • Cancer

KEY POINTS

- The success of precision medicine for humans is based on the understanding of cancer's great genomic heterogeneity and the successful pairing of therapies with the genomic mutations they target.
- Genomic changes shared between human and canine tumors have been the basis for predictions that human-approved drugs can be successfully used in canine oncology, and these hypotheses have shown early initial promise.
- Multiple genomic assays, spanning early cancer detection to treatment and monitoring, are currently available to all veterinarians.
- A growing body of information is available surrounding the safety and early efficacy of targeted therapeutics in dogs.

BACKGROUND
Human Precision Medicine

The human cancer precision medicine paradigm has been built on the foundation of understanding cancer's genomic underpinnings and great individual variability
Remarkable improvements in human cancer patient outcomes have been achieved in recent decades, progress best represented by the dramatic drop in cancer death rates. As of 2020, death rates have dropped by 33% relative to their peak in 1991, accounting for 3.8 million lives saved. This progress is due to improvements in treatment, early detection and diagnosis, and management of risk factors, all of which are components of the precision medicine paradigm arising over the past 30 years.[1] "Precision medicine" is defined by the National Institutes of Health's National Cancer Institute (NCI) as: "A form of medicine that uses information about a person's own genes or

[a] Vidium Animal Health, 7201 East Henkel Way, Suite 210, Scottsdale, AZ 85255, USA;
[b] OneHealthCompany, Inc, 530 Lytton Avenue, 2nd Floor, Palo Alto, CA 94301, USA
* Corresponding author.
E-mail address: gerry@fidocure.com

Vet Clin Small Anim 54 (2024) 501–521
https://doi.org/10.1016/j.cvsm.2023.12.006
0195-5616/24/© 2023 Elsevier Inc. All rights reserved.

vetsmall.theclinics.com

proteins to prevent, diagnose, or treat disease. In cancer, precision medicine uses specific information about a person's tumor to help make a diagnosis, plan treatment, find out how well treatment is working, or make a prognosis...".[2] A common misconception of cancer precision medicine dispelled by this definition is that precision medicine refers solely to the use of cancer gene sequencing tests to guide the selection of targeted treatments. Although this type of testing (cancer gene sequencing) and this use case for the testing (treatment guidance) are important examples of clinical tools and scenarios at the forefront of precision care delivery culminating from decades of research, they are only part of many aspects of the precision medicine approach. Critically important broader aspects of precision medicine in the NCI's definition include: (1) broader emphasis on uses of individual patient molecular information (whether genes, proteins, or other factors) to supplement what has historically been a more "one-size-fits-all" model focused on phenotypes (clinical signs, symptoms, imaging, and pathology), and (2) broader emphasis on not just use of molecular information for drug selection but also for guiding prevention, diagnosis, and prognostication.

The precision medicine paradigm not only includes clinical practice as emphasized in the NCI's definition but also translational research where it guides an improved understanding of tumor biology, tumor classification, and development of new drugs and diagnostics—all in the setting of individual patient variability and a molecular understanding of cancer in individual patients. The human cancer precision medicine paradigm has been built on the foundational recognition of cancer's genetic basis and our growing understanding of its vast and often subtly hidden individual variability.[3–5] Through a series of studies in human colorectal cancer more than 30 years ago that tracked the genetic progression of these tumors from adenomas to advanced metastatic disease, it became clear that cancer occurs when mutations in genes that regulate cell life, cell death, and cell:cell interactions accumulate clonally in expanding cell populations.[5] At the convergence of genetics, cell and functional biology, and clinical research, it then became clear that these cancer gene mutations give rise to aggressive cell- and tissue-level phenotypes, such as excessive growth or invasion, leading to the formation of malignant tumors that spread through tissues, organ systems, and entire organisms.[3] The background genetics and environment of the whole organism as well as the individual initiating cell in which these mutations arise can also alter the trajectory of developing cancers in different patients even though we often clinically observe relatively high levels of phenotypic convergence based on clinical presentation, imaging, and histology within individual tumor types.[4] The vast potential genomic variability hiding below the surface of any individual cancer diagnosis was first made clear in the mid-2000s after a revolution in DNA sequencing technology drove the cost and turnaround time of sequencing a single genome down from greater than $100M in years in 2000 to less than $1k and 24 hours today.[6] This allowed us to move from evaluating individual mutations in a handful of patients in the 1990s to characterizing entire genomes in thousands of patients today alongside deep analysis of many other molecules (eg, RNA, protein, epigenomic marks) and functional studies in tandem. These studies have reshaped our understanding of cancer by uncovering the great genomic complexity below the surface of any given tumor type.[7]

Milestones in the emergence of the human cancer precision medicine paradigm

Across the decades-long complex history of the rise of human cancer precision medicine, several milestones capture the major shifts in clinical practice and the research discoveries that drove them. First, emerging from genetic studies of whole chromosomes in the 1960s and 1970s was the discovery that some mutations were highly specific for individual cancer types (ie, diagnostic). These mutations also, by virtue of being necessary for both the initiation and ongoing survival of cancer cells, could potentially serve as drug targets unique to the cancer cells and thereby result in broad therapeutic windows and high response rates, in contrast to nonspecific effects of cytotoxic chemotherapy. The prototypical example is the discovery of the Philadelphia chromosome in chronic myelogenous leukemia (CML). This "chromosome" is a DNA translocation in which two separate chromosomes, 9 and 22, have broken and reassembled to create a new fusion gene, *BCR-ABL1*. The resulting protein is a constitutively active tyrosine kinase that drives excessive, malignant growth signaling. The *BCR-ABL1* translocation is highly sensitive and specific for CML diagnosis, occurring in most CML cases, and is regularly evaluated as part of the diagnostic workup. Drug studies culminated in the discovery in the mid-90s that the targeted small molecule tyrosine kinase inhibitor (TKI) imatinib (Gleevec) could selectively kill CML cells. Imatinib has since proven highly successful in treating CML patients.[8] These discoveries cemented the early recognition of the value of genetics in cancer diagnostics while also launching the targeted therapy paradigm that is a cornerstone of cancer precision medicine and, through many similar discoveries across many tumor types, has been enabling tailored cancer treatment based on the individual and not solely on histology.

The success of imatinib in CML brought hope at the turn of the millennium that new, tumor-type-specific drugs could be developed to exploit common vulnerabilities within certain histologies. This stimulated biology- and pathway-driven drug development programs associated with specific tumor types. However, cancer's genomic heterogeneity, even within tumor types, and its importance for drug design and treatment response were not yet fully appreciated until a second set of discoveries in the 2000s. These studies uncovered drug responses correlating with specific mutations that unlike *BCR-ABL1* in CML only occur in a subset of patients. Representative of these efforts were the parallel, but unique development paths for the targeted therapies gefitinib (Iressa, first-in-class epidermal growth factor receptor [EGFR] inhibitor) and vemurafenib (Zelboraf, first-in-class BRAF inhibitor). Gefitinib is a small molecule EGFR inhibitor that was originally developed agnostic to genetics and based instead on the recognition that EGFR is overexpressed in many human epithelial cancers including lung cancer. It was initially evaluated in unselected patient populations for patients with advanced non-small cell lung cancer (NSCLC). After receiving accelerated approval in 2003, it subsequently failed to show improved outcomes in confirmatory trials. Thus, AstraZeneca, the drug's manufacturer, agreed to withdraw the drug from the United States market. Meanwhile, genetic analyses in 2004 determined that constitutively activating *EGFR* mutations were present in ∼ 15% of Caucasian and 50% of Asian patients. This discovery led to new clinical trials that incorporated *EGFR*-mutant–patient subgroup analysis or stratification and the subsequent major finding of a greater than 50% response rate in *EGFR*-mutant patients alongside substantially longer progression-free survival (PFS) versus chemotherapy in the frontline setting. In 2015, gefitinib was then approved by the Food and Drug Administration (FDA) for the initial treatment of *EGFR*-mutant metastatic NSCLC alongside a companion diagnostic test for *EGFR* mutations.[9] Another example, in contrast to the *post hoc* rescue of gefitinib through genomic stratification, is that of vemurafenib, which was strategically developed in response to the 2002 discovery of activating *BRAF* mutations in ∼50% of metastatic cutaneous melanoma patients. Vemurafenib was the optimized result of a structure-guided drug design and discovery program aimed at disrupting mutated *BRAF*. Unlike gefitinib, it was specifically tested in *BRAF*-mutant melanoma patients where it was found to have a ∼50% response rate and to confer dramatic improvements in progression-free and overall survival relative to chemotherapy.[10] Since the early days of targeted and stratified drug development beginning with imatinib in 2001, more than 100 molecularly targeted anticancer agents have been approved by the FDA, many alongside companion diagnostics (including gene sequencing panels) for use in select patient populations within and even across tumor types.[11,12] This stratification has cemented the utility of thinking about cancer as a genetic disease that should be treated not just by tumor type but also individual genomic subtype.

The final milestone in the initial development of the human cancer precision medicine paradigm was the discovery of cancer's massive heterogeneity. As genomic sequencing technology became more accessible in the late 2000s, a growing number of individual research teams as well as multisite genomic consortia developed for the express purpose of harmonized genomic characterization of large cancer populations began to map the genomic landscapes of cancer ultimately across tens of thousands of patients with cancer.[7,13,14] Discoveries emerging from these studies revealed that cancer was far more complex than even early genomic studies had suggested, with most tumors bearing at least several driver mutations alongside dozens, hundreds, and, in some cases, even thousands of passenger mutations. Overall, more than 295,439 unique, likely pathogenic mutations in 707 cancer genes have been identified in more than 200 cancer types from hundreds of thousands of human cancer cases (COSMIC v95).[15] Although broad mutation patterns often track by tumor type, a large potential number of permutations of these mutations mean that most individual cancers bear a unique genomic signature. Yet, these mutations do often converge on shared pathways that intersect the large and growing list of targeted therapies. These mutations are increasingly well understood and many are associated with significant clinical value. More than 5000 mutation-based biomarkers are used in diagnosis, prognostication and/or therapy guidance in human cancer with ~1500 such mutations included in FDA or National Comprehensive Cancer Network clinical guidelines.[16–18] Thus, this understanding of cancer's substantial genomic variability along with recognition of the biomarker value of mutations and the potential for targeted therapies to improve outcomes in the setting of particular mutations together have established the precision medicine paradigm in which a cancer's genomic makeup must be considered in the care of the individual patient.

Human cancer precision medicine is improving patients' lives in routine practice today
The above discoveries reflect broader trends in human oncology research and clinical practice that have refined our understanding of cancer's initiation and progression while also shaping the development of new cancer treatments. At the same time, they have shaped the emergence of a thriving new discipline and diagnostic workstreams in human cancer medicine. Precision medicine is now an established tool that is a fundamental component not only of cancer research but also of daily, routine, clinical practice. For example, molecular pathology has rapidly grown over the past 25 years to focus on the incorporation of genomic and molecular information into clinical practice. In the United States, there are more than 231 boarded molecular pathologists, 1240 medical geneticists, and 2600 members of the American Association of Molecular Pathology.[19] In addition, more than 80 cancer genetics or genomics laboratories exist in the United States across academia and industry, offering more than 1500 cancer genetic or genomic assays that are used in clinical practice and approved by regulatory agencies.

Although there is a much wider world of cancer genomics research, drug development, and diagnostics that comprises cancer precision medicine as discussed earlier, the term "cancer precision medicine" is often associated specifically with the use of cancer gene sequencing panels that evaluate many genes and mutations at once, often in a pan-cancer setting and are regularly used to inform the management of human cancer patients (with many variations on when and how they are used). Questions about the value of such testing often center on cost, efficacy ("matching" and response rates), off-label drug use, and, in general, evidence to support the nonstandard decision-making that such tests can enable. Thus, many studies have sought to assess the clinical benefit of broad genomic profiling, typically for treatment selection in prospective clinical trials and often in pan-cancer settings, with well-known examples including the BATTLE, IMPACT, SHIVA, I-PREDICT, PERMED, and NCI MATCH studies.[20–24] Most of these studies show clear clinical benefit of some type, particularly in comparison to cytotoxic chemotherapy regimens. However, biomarker:drug match rates and response rates are sometimes low. These studies are often complex, nuanced, and challenging to interpret, particularly in regard to their real-world clinical value because they often focus on use in heavily pretreated cancer patients at academic centers and because, unlike in veterinary oncology, a robust standard of care exists for most human cancer patients and these patients also often have access to numerous clinical trials. However, evaluation of genomic diagnostic panels in real-world community hospital settings (ie, private hospital systems not affiliated with universities) has also been shown that they improve outcomes while reducing treatment costs and improving quality of life.[25,26] Meanwhile, a significant ongoing need exists for identification of new genomic biomarkers, development of new effective therapeutics alongside companion diagnostics to facilitate their use in high-impact settings, and continuing refinement of incorporation of genomic diagnostics into the clinical care stream.

Summary
Genomics and precision medicine are not only driving the leading edge of care but are also inextricably woven into the standard of care for most human cancer patients today. Advances in the genomic understanding of human cancer have been steadily bringing new and powerful tools to the human cancer clinic since the 1970s including new diagnostics (single cancer genes/mutations, cancer gene panels, and companion diagnostics) and new drugs, many of which are now developed in a genomically stratified setting. In veterinary oncology, although limited by dramatically fewer resources, we are increasingly equipped to bring this innovation to the care of pets with cancer both via inference and lessons learned from human cancer precision medicine as well as through growing progress being made directly in canine cancer research.

Veterinary Precision Medicine
Veterinarians have a long history of using precision medicine for purebred dogs using breed as a proxy for certain clinically relevant genotypes in many situations including interpretation of diagnostics (eg, hematocrit in greyhounds[27]), recommendations for screening (eg, presurgical coagulation screening in Doberman Pinschers[28]), and drug choices (eg, caution with ivermectin in collies[29]). A major breakthrough for veterinary precision medicine was made possible with the publication of the first canine reference genome in 2005 by Lindblad-Toh and colleagues. This resource represents a significant milestone in veterinary and comparative medicine,[30] enabling the identification and characterization of canine genomic alterations, including disease-associated mutations, structural variants, and regulatory elements. Among these subsequent discoveries have been cancer-associated genomic variants and molecular markers.[31–35]

These studies have shed light on the underlying genomic alterations and molecular pathways that drive canine cancers, providing valuable insights into tumor development and progression. By identifying specific genomic mutations, chromosomal abnormalities, and gene expression patterns particular to specific cancers, researchers have begun to characterize molecular signatures for some canine tumors.[36,37] Genomic and molecular knowledge has paved the way for developing diagnostic tools and targeted therapies.[38–42] Although the first version of the feline reference genome was published 1 year after its canine counterpart,[43] this draft was low coverage (2X) and highly fragmented. Relative to the dog genome, slow progress in the improvement and annotation of the feline genome from 2006 to 2020[44] has further delayed the potential applications of cancer genomics for this species.[45]

In dogs, the genetic diversity that exists across the entire genome is comparable to that across the human genome and thus expectations that certain targeted therapies may work in specific subpopulations of patients even in cases of poor overall drug efficacy in clinical trials is as valid in canine patients as it is for humans. Indeed, there may be greater hope for such successes in canine subpopulations because of the unique population structure of domestic dogs, with the overall diversity being siloed within breeds[46,47] and thus, even in mixed breed dogs, inherited according to recent breed ancestry. In other words, there is good reason to expect that a drug showing efficacy in only a small percentage of dogs in a genetically diverse canine clinical trial cohort or even no efficacy in a genetically homogenous canine clinical trial (eg, a single breed group) may prove extremely efficacious in a population enriched for a certain biomarker or shared ancestry.

Precision medicine and genetic tests for dogs with cancer

Advances in genomic characterization of tumors are crucial for the implementation of precision medicine approaches to treat cancer in dogs. The molecular phenotyping of canine tumors has revealed striking similarities to those characteristics identified in humans, enabling translation of knowledge and therapeutic strategies from human medicine to veterinary oncology. As a result, precision treatments that have proven effective in human patients are now being adapted and used in dogs, enhancing their chances of successful treatment outcomes,[40] advancing our understanding of cancer biology, improving treatment options for both species,[48] and offering the potential to streamline cancer drug development pipelines.[49] However, significant challenges still arise from the limited genomic information available for certain canine tumor types, limiting the possibility of comparative precision medicine trials. Representative genetic profiles of cancer types such as thyroid carcinoma, anal sac adenocarcinoma, neuroendocrine tumors, and others have been published only recently,[35] and many more studies of various cancer types are needed.

As genomic research is completed, the implementation of precision medicine can be accelerated in veterinary medicine compared with human medicine because of the relative paucity of regulations in veterinary medicine.[50,51] This increased flexibility in veterinary medicine increases the number of options available for pets in terms of treatment, including deviations from typical "first-line" protocols, off-label drug uses, and drug combinations.

Technological advancements facilitated the development of specific diagnostic tests, such as the identification of the V595E mutation of the *BRAF* gene in DNA found in the urine of dogs with urothelial carcinoma or transitional cell carcinoma. *BRAF* V595E has been identified in 75% to 80% of dogs with urothelial carcinoma[38,39] and can be identified in urine and bladder biopsies in the early stage of disease and thus allow faster accurate diagnosis of affected dogs.[52]

Continued advancements have led to development of several next-generation sequencing (NGS) assays in veterinary medicine,[53–55] two of which are currently commercially available. These genomic tests can be performed using DNA from formalin-fixed paraffin-embedded (FFPE) tissue or fine-needle aspirates (FNAs) facilitating their incorporation into clinical routines. In 2019 and 2020, the One Health Company and Vidium Animal Health launched FidoCure and SearchLight DNA, respectively. Both assays, available for the veterinary community, harness the power of NGS platforms to create comprehensive genomic profiles of canine cancers, facilitating the identification of mutated oncogenes and tumor suppressor genes in canine cancer and enabling genomic-guided small-molecule targeted therapy.

Recently, circulating cell-free DNA (cfDNA) has been used for cancer diagnosis in dogs. cfDNA refers to small fragments of DNA that circulate in the plasma. These fragments are released during the turnover of apoptotic and necrotic cells, including both normal and cancer cells.[56] cfDNA is typically found at lower levels in healthy patients and higher levels in patients with cancer. In veterinary medicine, various approaches involving cfDNA have been investigated. For instance, researchers have explored the measurement of cfDNA concentration to assess prognosis of dogs with cancer.[57–59] Small genomic alterations have been detected from DNA in plasma from dogs with cancer using polymerase chain reaction (PCR),[60] and NGS has enabled the identification of different types of genomic alterations that, in combination with bioinformatic algorithms, can detect cancer in dogs with an overall sensitivity across all cancer-diagnosed dogs of 54.7%.[61] The utility of cfDNA has been evaluated in different aspects of clinical oncology for different tumor types. Measurement of cfDNA associated with DNA integrity index using fragments of long interspersed nuclear element-1 is a valuable biomarker for disease progression monitoring in dogs with oral malignant melanoma.[62] Another non-genomic (nucleosome-based) liquid biopsy assay is also commercially available.[63] Liquid biopsy has provided valuable insights for not only cancer diagnosis but also therapy selection, treatment response, and disease monitoring.[64,65] Genomic characterization enables identification of specific genetic alterations that guide targeted therapy selection. It allows clinicians to tailor therapies to the unique genomic profile of the tumor, enhancing treatment efficacy and minimizing unnecessary side effects.[66,67]

Targeted therapy in dogs with cancer

Several different types of targeted therapies are currently used in veterinary medicine, including small molecule inhibitors and monoclonal antibodies (mABs). Small molecule inhibitors cause a direct effect on tumor cells, competitively inhibiting receptors in a reversible or irreversible manner. A major category of small molecule inhibitors in veterinary medicine are those inhibiting tyrosine kinases (mediators of signaling pathways of cell proliferation, differentiation, migration, angiogenesis, and cell-cycle regulation). TKIs effectively hinder the kinase's ability to phosphorylate itself and initiate downstream signaling cascades.[68,69] To ensure selectivity for specific proteins, researchers have extensively characterized the adenosine triphosphate (ATP)-binding pockets of various kinases. This knowledge enables design of inhibitors exhibiting activity against restricted subsets of kinases, thereby minimizing off-target effects on non-targeted kinases. These inhibitors are often amenable to large-scale synthesis, possess oral bioavailability, and readily penetrate cells to reach their intended targets. Toceranib phosphate (Palladia, Zoetis) and masitinib (Masivet, AB Science) were the first TKIs approved by the FDA and the European Medicine Agency, respectively, for dogs with mast cell tumors (MCTs). These small molecules have potent inhibitory activity against members of the kinase receptor families such as VEGFR, PDGFR, RET, and Kit, resulting in antitumor and antiangiogenic effects.[70,71]

Small molecules can block specific pathways related to carcinogenesis, tumor growth and block specific enzymes, growth factors, and receptors responsible for cell proliferation.[72] Small molecules are commonly recommended for human cancer treatment, usually when a specific target is identified from NGS-based companion diagnostics that inform who could benefit from this specific treatment. This precision medicine approach has already been used to treat canine cancers.[40] Because there is an overlap of 50 well-known oncogene and tumor suppressor genes, including hotspot mutations between both species,[35] treatment using small molecules guided by genetic alterations are likely to also bring benefits for dogs with cancer.

Instead of having a direct effect on tumor cell activity, mABs are engineered to bind to specific proteins on the cancer cells and have unique immune-effector mechanisms, such as antibody-dependent cellular toxicity, complement-dependent cytotoxicity, and complement-dependent cell-mediated cytotoxicity.[73] Unfortunately, clinical trials assessing the efficacy of two caninized mABs developed by Aratana Pharmaceuticals for the treatment of B-cell and T-cell canine lymphoma, respectively, have yielded disappointing results, potentially because of nonspecific binding activities of these antibodies.[74] On the other hand, the immune checkpoint blocking programmed cell death 1 has been under investigation with promising results both in vitro and in vivo,[75–78] especially for melanomas,[79,80] and anal sac adenocarcinoma.[81]

The use of small molecules and mABs to treat cancer in dogs provides an opportunity for bespoke and targeted treatments that are tumor-specific rather than delivering systemic toxic chemotherapies to deplete all rapidly dividing cells. Because of the paucity of veterinary-approved small molecules available and the fact that veterinarians can legally use drugs approved for human use as long as there is no commercially available veterinary equivalent, human small molecule therapies have been used with the outcomes reported in the literature. For example, in canine transitional cell carcinoma, dysregulation in the EGFR signaling pathways is present in the majority of cases. As no veterinary-specific EGFR inhibitor is approved, the human-approved EGFR inhibitor, lapatinib, has been used off-label and shown efficacy in treating this disease.[41]

Precision medicine approaches have not just been used to improve companion animal care. Genomic data associated with proteomic, transcriptomic, and metabolomic data have been used as important tools in conservation medicine as they do not require species-specific diagnostic tests. Hypotheses can be examined and validated through computational approaches without being constrained by the availability of additional samples. Whilde and colleagues discussed several case studies where precision medicine was used to help with conditions affecting threatened species including fibropapillomatosis in sea turtles, tumors in beluga whales, Ebola virus in African great apes, chytridiomycosis in amphibians, and facial tumor disease in Tasmanian devils.[82]

Overall, precision medicine has the potential to revolutionize the way we diagnose and treat canine cancer. Although much more research is needed in this area, early results are promising, and it is likely that precision medicine will play an increasingly important role in veterinary oncology in the years to come.

DISCUSSION
Guidelines

WHY would one consider precision medicine for the canine cancer patient?
The genomic homology between people and dogs lends support to the same success of precision medicine in dogs as it has in people. The utilization of an individual's cancer genomic signature for the selection of specific targeted therapies has proven successful in human oncology, improving outcomes and quality of life for patients with cancer.[9–12,25,26] Shared molecular mechanisms between dogs and humans, along

with orthologous genomic alterations in cancer genes affecting corresponding biological pathways, support the potential benefit of using human genomic information for clinical inferences in dogs.[48,49] In fact, the structured analysis of sequence conservation and conversion of human mutations to the canine genome ("caninisation") has recently been applied to COSMIC, the most prominent human cancer mutation database, identifying shared putative cancer-driving mutations and mutations bearing similar biomarker associations with diagnostic, prognostic, and therapeutic utility.[83] This structured caninization of human cancer mutations facilitates the interpretation and annotation of canine mutations, allowing for the reasonable inference of mutation-based biomarker data from the information-rich human oncology space and responsibly meeting the clinical needs of canine cancer patients.

Precision medicine is widely available for dogs, with utility in all steps of the cancer journey. There is already emerging evidence of precision medicine's clinical benefit in dogs. By leveraging the caninization of the abundant human mutation-based biomarker information, genomic testing in dogs has demonstrated utility in providing diagnostic guidance, prognostic support, and therapeutic options for canine cancer patients, particularly those that have ambiguous diagnoses and therefore are inherently challenging to manage.[84] A recent real-world clinicogenomics study unveiled gene-level prognostic indications for several cancer genes and potential association of mutant genes with response to targeted therapies.[40] A separate study identified novel mutations with prognostic value and demonstrated the benefit of targeted therapies, particularly those that are genomically informed, across multiple cancer types in dogs.[85] This therapeutic utility of genomic analysis allows for more effective clinical decision-making for treatment interventions with targeted therapeutics that could eventually prove to have synergy with or even superiority over conventional therapies. Another meaningful avenue of genomics is screening for early cancer detection and for cancer monitoring. An NGS-based liquid biopsy technique has demonstrated utility as a novel option for noninvasive multi-cancer detection in dogs.[61,86,87] In their entirety, these bodies of work provide a compelling view of the significant potential in genomics and precision medicine for dogs with cancer. Resulting genomic and outcome data gathered from these genomic analyses could then feed back into a data pool that could ultimately guide novel drug development for dogs and people with cancer.

Owing to the heterogeneity of cancer, there is a need for individualized testing. The explosion of molecular technology has highlighted the inter- and intra-tumoral heterogeneity within cancer types as well as across different cancers in both dogs and people.[88–90] Appreciation of this genomic diversity calls for individualized testing using diagnostic assays to characterize a broad range of cancer types. For people, as more molecularly guided treatments become FDA-approved, companion diagnostics are developed alongside them to inform selection of patients for these targeted approaches. In veterinary medicine, fewer though still highly impactful assays are increasingly available and easily accessible, enabling our canine patients to shift away from the "one-size-fits-all" therapeutic paradigm to one that is more personalized and biomarker-guided.

WHAT genomic tests are currently available for dogs?
Multiple precision medicine tools are already commercially available and increasingly used in dogs. For dogs with cancer, there are currently several genomic assays available. Two of these use NGS technology to simultaneously evaluate multiple mutation types in multiple genes across a variety of cancers. SearchLight DNA (Vidium Animal Health) identifies copy number variants, single-nucleotide variants, and internal

tandem duplications in 120 cancer genes. Mutations are then annotated as biomarkers of diagnosis, prognosis, and therapy, with supporting evidence levels from published literature for each biomarker association. Fidocure (The One Health Company) sequences the entire coding region of 56 commonly mutated cancer genes, identifying single-nucleotide variants, insertions and deletions, and copy number variants. Mutations identified in each patient and the relevant scientific evidence for each variant's relevance for prognosis and therapy guidance are described in a unique patient report, and therapies can be ordered and delivered to the patient's home through Fidocure's partner compounding pharmacies.

There are several other tests that are focused on evaluating one or two genes for specific cancers, using the PCR method. PARR (PCR for antigen receptor rearrangements; offered by multiple institutions and companies) evaluates clonality of T-cell receptor and/or immunoglobulin heavy chain genes to immunophenotype and/or distinguish lymphoproliferative neoplasia from inflammation. Other available tests include C-kit PCR (for internal tandem duplication mutation in exon 8 and/or exon 11 in the c-kit gene; Michigan State University [MSU]); PTPN11 mutation PCR (for E76K substitution mutation in the PTPN11 gene; MSU); transmissible venereal tumor (TVT) PCR (for long interspersed elements in the cellular myelocytomatosis oncogene [c-MYC] gene; MSU); CADET *BRAF* and CADET *BRAF-PLUS* (for V595E and copy number mutations in the BRAF gene; Antech) to aide in the diagnosis of MCT/gastrointestinal stromal tumor (GIST), melanoma, histiocytic sarcoma, TVT, and urothelial carcinoma, respectively.

For early cancer detection in dogs, OncoK9 (PetDx) is a genomic screening test that uses the liquid biopsy method. OncoK9 detects cfDNA—specifically a fraction of cfDNA called the circulating tumor DNA (ctDNA) that originates from tumor cells—via NGS. A clinical validation study demonstrated this assay's detection of cancer signal in patients representing 30 distinct cancer types.[61]

WHEN should one consider precision medicine?
There are many clinical scenarios where precision medicine tools should be considered for dogs: diagnostic guidance, prognostication, therapeutic options, cancer screening, and cancer monitoring. *Diagnosis*: Genomic tests that are already commonly used in the diagnostic setting are the PCR-based tests (CADET *BRAF*, PARR, and so forth). These tests aid in the diagnosis of specific cancers if they are highly suspected from first-line pathologic evaluation. SearchLight DNA, an NGS-based assay, can also be used for diagnostic clarification[84] in cases that are diagnostically ambiguous, based on annotation of identified mutations using human consensus guidelines.

Prognosis: Cancer prognostication can be performed with both SearchLight DNA and Fidocure. For SearchLight DNA, the same process that is used to annotate diagnostic and therapeutic biomarkers is also used to annotate identified mutations as prognostic. A recent study that used SearchLight DNA identified six genes that were associated with shorter PFS. This same study also revealed genomically informed targeted therapy given before first progression was associated with a significantly longer PFS (submitted for publication). Another study that used Fidocure identified five genes associated with either a positive or negative prognosis.[40]

Therapy: Both SearchLight DNA and Fidocure can also be used for therapeutic guidance. These assays identify mutations that are associated with response to targeted therapies based on published studies that range from preclinical in vitro studies to well-powered in vivo studies validating mutations as proven therapeutic biomarkers. Genomically guided therapies can be used in addition to, in combination with, or in lieu of conventional therapies, depending on the aggressiveness of the patient's cancer, owner's wishes, and/or clinician's professional guidance.

Screening: OncoK9 is a multi-cancer early detection test for the detection and characterization of cancer-associated genomic alterations. It is intended for use in dogs that are at higher risk of cancer.

Application

HOW does one apply these tests in practice?
Case selection: Any cases that are at risk of developing cancer (such as older dogs and/or predisposed breeds) could benefit from early screening before the development of clinical signs. For diagnostic elucidation, cases that remain equivocal after initial pathologic (cytologic or histologic) evaluation could benefit from PCR tests that specifically evaluate cancers on the list of differential diagnoses and/or from SearchLight DNA. Uncommon cases or cases that do not have definitive diagnoses could also benefit from SearchLight DNA or Fidocure, which can provide prognostic information based on the identification of mutations in specific prognostic genes. Dogs that need more aggressive therapy or have failed or cannot receive conventional therapy should also consider SearchLight DNA and Fidocure for selection of targeted therapeutic options.

Sample types and unique collection methods: PARR can be performed from either FFPE tissues or aspirates (depending on the providing company or institution). PCR for c-MYC mutation (to evaluate for TVT) and C-kit mutation (to evaluate for MCT/GIST/melanoma) can be performed on FFPE/formalin-fixed/fresh tissues or aspirates. PCR for PTPN11 mutation (to evaluate for histiocytic sarcoma) requires whole blood in ethylenediaminetetraacetic acid (EDTA) tubes. PCR for BRAF mutation (to evaluate for urothelial carcinomas) requires a free-caught urine sample into a dedicated CADET *BRAF* urine specimen container that contains a stabilizing agent. OncoK9 requires a peripheral whole blood sample that is collected into specialized blood collection tubes designed to prevent white blood cell lysis and cfDNA degradation. Fidocure is performed on FFPE samples. SearchLight DNA can be performed on FFPE tissue, FNAs, and most sample types in which sufficient neoplastic cellularity can be confirmed by internal pathology review, such as spun-down urine and effusions, on a case-by-case basis.

WHO can use these tests?
All veterinarians, including but not limited to those involved with primary care, emergency care, shelter medicine, and specialty care, have equal and easy access to all genomic assays.

For WHAT cancers should these tests be performed?
Because the purpose of the PCR-based tests is to facilitate differentiation of cancer types that may be morphologically difficult to distinguish, these tests should be considered after the differential diagnoses have been narrowed to include the cancer types for which the PCR assay is proposed to facilitate in diagnosing. SearchLight DNA and Fidocure are designed to include all cancer types and can therefore be performed on all cancers for which the sample type is accepted.

Therapeutic Options Guided by Genomic Analysis

Multiple targeted therapeutics, for which there are pharmacokinetic and safety data, are currently available to veterinarians from at least one major compounding pharmacy in the United States (**Table 1**).

Limitations

There are potential limitations to these assays. By only evaluating one or two genes in the PCR-based assays, we may be missing other critical genes that could have

Table 1
Targeted therapies currently available for dogs

Targeted Therapy	Suggested NOAEL[a]	Typical Starting Dose[b]	Possible Clinical Signs[c]	Notable Laboratory Abnormalities[d]	Availability to Veterinarians[e]	Availability of Pharmacokinetic Data
Crizotinib	<5 mg/kg/day	1–2 mg/kg/day	Emesis; watery/mucoid feces	CBC (decreased RBC parameters; increased WBC parameters; increased platelets). Serum biochemistry (increased ALT, AST, ALP, GGT; decreased albumin and calcium)	Yes	Yes
Dasatinib	<0.75 mg/kg/day	0.5 mg/kg/day	Emesis and bloody vomitus; liquid, mucous, and blood in feces	Serum biochemistry (decreased total protein, albumin, globulins; increased ALT)	Yes	Yes
Ibrutinib	1.5 mg/kg/day	2.5–5 mg/kg/day	Soft feces/diarrhea; emesis; decreased food consumption; reddened or pale gums; raised reddened or white areas on gums; tremors; intermittent convulsion, rigid muscle tone	CBC (increased WBC parameters; increased platelets). Serum biochemistry (increased AST, triglycerides)	Yes	Yes
Imatinib	3 mg/kg/day	10 mg/kg/day	Emesis	CBC (decreased RBC and WBC parameters). Serum biochemistry (increased ALT)	Yes	Yes
Lapatinib	10 mg/kg/day	20–30 mg/kg/day	Decreased activity; dehydration; salivation; loose feces; ulcerations in paw and mouth; scabs; emesis	CBC (increased WBC parameters). Serum biochemistry (increased bilirubin, total bile acids, ALP, ALT). Urinalysis (increased bilirubin)	Yes	Yes

Drug	Dose	Dose	Clinical signs	Laboratory changes		
Olaparib	<3 mg/kg/day	2.5–3 mg/kg/day	Lethargy	CBC (decreased RBC and WBC parameters; decreased platelets)	Yes	Yes
Palbociclib	<2 mg/kg/day	0.6 mg/kg/day	Soft feces; red/swollen pinnae	CBC (decreased RBC and WBC parameters, particularly neutrophils; decreased platelets)	Yes	Yes
Sirolimus	<0.1 mg/kg/day	0.1 mg/kg/day	Emesis; diarrhea; anorexia; weight loss; red lesions on gums	CBC (increased WBC parameters)	Yes	Yes
Sorafenib	<3 mg/kg/day	5 mg/kg q12 h	Liquid feces ± blood or mucus; weight loss; sparse hair coat, pustules, alopecia with reddened or bluish skin, dark axillary skin	CBC (decreased RBC parameters; increased WBC parameters; increased platelets). Serum biochemistry (increased ALT, AST, ALP, GGT)	Yes	Yes
Toceranib	Not observed (clinical changes noted at all evaluated dose levels)	2.75 mg/kg every other day	Diarrhea, blood in stool, hemorrhagic diarrhea; anorexia; lethargy; vomiting; nausea; lameness; weight loss; dermatitis; pruritus; tachypnea; localized pain; flatulence; conjunctivitis	CBC (decreased hematocrit; decreased platelets; decreased neutrophils). Serum biochemistry (increased ALT, creatinine, bilirubin; decreased albumin). Urinalysis (urinary tract infection)	Yes	Yes
Trametinib	<0.4 mg/m^2/day	0.5 mg/m^2/day	Skin lesions, scabs, discharge from and swelling of prepuce or vulva; salivation; gastrointestinal toxicity; lethargy	CBC (anemia, increased reticulocyte count). Serum biochemistry (increased liver enzymes). Urinalysis and/or UPC (increased protein). Blood pressure (increased)	Yes	Yes

(continued on next page)

Table 1
(continued)

Targeted Therapy	Suggested NOAEL[a]	Typical Starting Dose[b]	Possible Clinical Signs[c]	Notable Laboratory Abnormalities[d]	Availability to Veterinarians[e]	Availability of Pharmacokinetic Data
Vorinostat	60 mg/kg/day	22 mg/kg every other day to 30 mg/kg/day	Non-formed or liquid feces; weight loss; dehydration; hypoactive behavior; pale gums; emesis; nausea	CBC (increased or decreased RBC parameters; increased WBC parameters; increased platelets). Serum biochemistry (increased APTT, protein, albumin, creatinine, BUN, BG; decreased P, Na, K, Cl). Urinalysis (increased urine volume, decreased USG, positive occult blood in urine)	Yes	Yes

Abbreviations: ALT, alanine transaminase; ALP, alkaline phosphatase; APTT, activated partial thromboplastin clotting time; AST, aspartate aminotransferase; BG, blood glucose; BUN, blood urea nitrogen; CBC, complete blood count; GGT, gamma-glutamyl transferase; RBC, red blood cell; NDA, new drug application; UPC, urine protein-to-creatinine ratio; USG, urine specific gravity; WBC, white blood cell.

[a] No observed adverse effect level, based on a combination of primary canine publications and canine-specific data in the NDA.
[b] Based on personal communication with multiple veterinary oncologists.
[c] Typically seen at doses significantly higher than NOAEL based on studies performed in the NDA, and these signs could also represent feedback from clinicians using this drug on their patients.
[d] Changes typically seen at doses higher than NOAEL.
[e] Available in at least one major compounding pharmacy in the United States.
Data from Refs.[91–104]

therapeutic, diagnostic, or prognostic biomarker associations. For pan-cancer, multi-gene panels, intra-tumoral heterogeneity may preclude representative sampling for genomic analysis. The efficacy of targeted therapeutics for dogs, whether used alone or in combination with conventional therapies, has yet to be fully explored, although we have early compelling evidence supporting its utility. Finally, for liquid biopsy methods that rely on ctDNA, there is a possibility for insufficient ctDNA in circulation for confident detection and characterization of cancer.

Looking Toward the Future

Emerging evidence of human precision medicine success paves a path toward its broad applications in veterinary medicine. There are already promising early indications for the utility of genomics in cancer monitoring via a noninvasive liquid biopsy method. Genomics can be used to predict future cancer development or to predict disease risk, such as the use of germline BRCA mutations to predict breast cancer risk in women. Genomics can also synergize with and mutually bolster other disciplines, such as immunotherapy, pharmacology, and other "'omics", providing a more comprehensive approach to cancer care. Finally, because sequencing technology continues to advance and become more efficient, we can expect the cost of performing high-throughput genomics to decline with time, allowing more pets to enjoy the many life-saving benefits of precision medicine.

SUMMARY

1. Precision medicine focuses on the clinical management of the patient based on the individual, not based on population-based findings.
2. There are many successes of precision medicine implementation in human oncology and it is therefore integrated into human cancer management. It is increasingly integrated into canine cancer management, with early evidence of its success.
3. In canine oncology, precision medicine can be integrated into practice as a complement to the conventional approaches to disease characterization, treatment, and monitoring.
4. As genomic profiling costs decrease with time, test costs will decrease, allowing for increased utilization and subsequent improvement of knowledge base from which to make better-informed decisions.
5. Integration of precision medicine in canine oncology has already begun and will only expand in utility and use by veterinarians for improved cancer characterization, enhanced therapy selection, and overall more successful management of canine cancer. As such, practitioners are called to interpret and leverage precision medicine reports for their patients.

CLINICS CARE POINTS

- Genomics-informed targeted therapies have proven repeatedly successful for human genomic targets, with initial evidence of efficacy in homologous canine targets.
- Several genomic assays, spanning cancer screening to treatment selection, are currently commercially available at the disposal of every veterinarian.
- A growing body of information is available surrounding the safety and early efficacy of targeted therapeutics in dogs.

DISCLOSURE

W. Hendricks is a full-time employee of Vidium Animal Health; E. Chon and D. Haworth were full time employees of Vidium Animal Health; SearchLight DNA is a product developed and provided by Vidium Animal Health. L. Rodrigues, and G. Post are full-time employees of One Health Company; M. White was a full time employee of One Health Company; FidoCure is a product developed and provided by One Health Company.

REFERENCES

1. American cancer society. American Cancer Society | Cancer Facts & Statistics Available at: http://cancerstatisticscenter.cancer.org. Accessed August 7, 2023.
2. Comprehensive cancer information. National Cancer Institute. 1980 Available at: http://www.cancer.gov. Accessed August 7, 2023.
3. Hanahan D, Weinberg RA. Hallmarks of cancer: the next generation. Cell 2011; 144(5):646–74.
4. Hanahan D. Hallmarks of Cancer: New Dimensions. Cancer Discov 2022;12(1): 31–46.
5. Fearon ER, Vogelstein B. A genetic model for colorectal tumorigenesis. Cell 1990;61(5):759–67.
6. About genomics. Genome.gov Available at: http://www.genome.gov/about-genomics. Accessed August 7, 2023.
7. Vogelstein B, Papadopoulos N, Velculescu VE, et al. Cancer genome landscapes. Science 2013;339(6127):1546–58.
8. Ren R. Mechanisms of BCR-ABL in the pathogenesis of chronic myelogenous leukaemia. Nat Rev Cancer 2005;5(3):172–83.
9. Rawluk J, Waller CF. Gefitinib. Recent Results Cancer Res 2018;211:235–46.
10. Flaherty KT, Yasothan U, Kirkpatrick P. Vemurafenib. Nat Rev Drug Discov 2011; 10(11):811–2.
11. Min HY, Lee HY. Molecular targeted therapy for anticancer treatment. Exp Mol Med 2022;54(10):1670–94.
12. Mateo J, Steuten L, Aftimos P, et al. Delivering precision oncology to patients with cancer. Nat Med 2022;28(4):658–65.
13. Cancer Genome Atlas Research Network, Weinstein JN, Collisson EA, et al. The Cancer Genome Atlas Pan-Cancer analysis project. Nat Genet 2013;45(10): 1113–20.
14. International Cancer Genome Consortium, Hudson TJ, Anderson W, et al. International network of cancer genome projects. Nature 2010;464(7291):993–8.
15. Forbes SA, Beare D, Boutselakis H, et al. COSMIC: somatic cancer genetics at high-resolution. Nucleic Acids Res 2017;45(D1):D777–83.
16. Chakravarty D, Gao J, Phillips SM, et al. OncoKB: A Precision Oncology Knowledge Base. JCO Precis Oncol 2017;2017. https://doi.org/10.1200/PO.17.00011.
17. Tamborero D, Rubio-Perez C, Deu-Pons J, et al. Cancer Genome Interpreter annotates the biological and clinical relevance of tumor alterations. Genome Med 2018;10(1):25.
18. Li MM, Datto M, Duncavage EJ, et al. Standards and Guidelines for the Interpretation and Reporting of Sequence Variants in Cancer: A Joint Consensus Recommendation of the Association for Molecular Pathology, American Society of Clinical Oncology, and College of American Pathologists. J Mol Diagn 2017; 19(1):4–23.

19. Home. Association for Molecular Pathology Available at: http://www.amp.org. Accessed August 7, 2023.

20. Kim ES, Herbst RS, Wistuba II, et al. The BATTLE trial: personalizing therapy for lung cancer. Cancer Discov 2011;1(1):44–53.

21. Tsimberidou AM, Hong DS, Ye Y, et al. Initiative for Molecular Profiling and Advanced Cancer Therapy (IMPACT): An MD Anderson Precision Medicine Study. JCO Precis Oncol 2017;2017. https://doi.org/10.1200/PO.17.00002.

22. Belin L, Kamal M, Mauborgne C, et al. Randomized phase II trial comparing molecularly targeted therapy based on tumor molecular profiling versus conventional therapy in patients with refractory cancer: cross-over analysis from the SHIVA trial. Ann Oncol 2017;28(3):590–6.

23. Sicklick JK, Kato S, Okamura R, et al. Molecular profiling of cancer patients enables personalized combination therapy: the I-PREDICT study. Nat Med 2019; 25(5):744–50.

24. Bertucci F, Gonçalves A, Guille A, et al. Prospective high-throughput genome profiling of advanced cancers: results of the PERMED-01 clinical trial. Genome Med 2021;13(1):87.

25. Haslem DS, Van Norman SB, Fulde G, et al. A Retrospective Analysis of Precision Medicine Outcomes in Patients With Advanced Cancer Reveals Improved Progression-Free Survival Without Increased Health Care Costs. J Oncol Pract 2017;13(2):e108–19.

26. Haslem DS, Chakravarty I, Fulde G, et al. Precision oncology in advanced cancer patients improves overall survival with lower weekly healthcare costs. Oncotarget 2018;9(15):12316–22.

27. Shiel RE, Brennan SF, O'Rourke LG, et al. Hematologic values in young pretraining healthy Greyhounds. Vet Clin Pathol 2007;36(3):274–7.

28. Johnstone IB. Canine Von Willebrand's Disease: A Common Inherited Bleeding Disorder in Doberman Pinscher Dogs. Can Vet J 1986;27(9):315–8.

29. Paul AJ, Tranquilli WJ, Seward RL, et al. Clinical observations in collies given ivermectin orally. Am J Vet Res 1987;48(4):684–5.

30. Lindblad-Toh K, Wade CM, Mikkelsen TS, et al. Genome sequence, comparative analysis and haplotype structure of the domestic dog. Nature 2005;438(7069): 803–19.

31. Simpson S, Dunning MD, de Brot S, et al. Comparative review of human and canine osteosarcoma: morphology, epidemiology, prognosis, treatment and genetics. Acta Vet Scand 2017;59(1):71.

32. Bergholtz H, Lien T, Lingaas F, et al. Comparative analysis of the molecular subtype landscape in canine and human mammary gland tumors. J Mammary Gland Biol Neoplasia 2022;27(2):171–83.

33. Hernandez B, Adissu HA, Wei BR, et al. Naturally Occurring Canine Melanoma as a Predictive Comparative Oncology Model for Human Mucosal and Other Triple Wild-Type Melanomas. Int J Mol Sci 2018;19(2). https://doi.org/10.3390/ijms19020394.

34. Wong S, Ehrhart EJ, Stewart S, et al. Genomic landscapes of canine splenic angiosarcoma (hemangiosarcoma) contain extensive heterogeneity within and between patients. PLoS One 2022;17(7):e0264986.

35. Rodrigues L, Watson J, Feng Y, et al. Shared hotspot mutations in oncogenes position dogs as an unparalleled comparative model for precision therapeutics. Sci Rep 2023;13(1):10935.

36. Wang G, Wu M, Maloneyhuss MA, et al. Actionable mutations in canine hemangiosarcoma. PLoS One 2017;12(11):e0188667.

37. Cronise KE, Das S, Hernandez BG, et al. Characterizing the molecular and immune landscape of canine bladder cancer. Vet Comp Oncol 2022;20(1):69–81.
38. Mochizuki H, Shapiro SG, Breen M. Detection of BRAF Mutation in Urine DNA as a Molecular Diagnostic for Canine Urothelial and Prostatic Carcinoma. PLoS One 2015;10(12):e0144170.
39. Decker B, Parker HG, Dhawan D, et al. Homologous mutation to human BRAF V600E is common in naturally occurring canine bladder cancer—Evidence for a relevant model system and urine-based diagnostic test. Mol Cancer Res 2015;13(6):993–1002.
40. Wu K, Rodrigues L, Post G, et al. Analyses of canine cancer mutations and treatment outcomes using real-world clinico-genomics data of 2119 dogs. npj Precis Oncol 2023;7(1):8.
41. Maeda S, Sakai K, Kaji K, et al. Lapatinib as first-line treatment for muscle-invasive urothelial carcinoma in dogs. Sci Rep 2022;12(1):4.
42. Paoloni MC, Mazcko C, Fox E, et al. Rapamycin pharmacokinetic and pharmacodynamic relationships in osteosarcoma: a comparative oncology study in dogs. PLoS One 2010;5(6):e11013.
43. JU Pontius, Mullikin JC, Smith DR, et al. Initial sequence and comparative analysis of the cat genome. Genome Res 2007;17(11):1675–89.
44. Buckley RM, Davis BW, Brashear WA, et al. A new domestic cat genome assembly based on long sequence reads empowers feline genomic medicine and identifies a novel gene for dwarfism. PLoS Genet 2020;16(10):e1008926.
45. Ludwig L, Dobromylskyj M, Wood GA, et al. Feline Oncogenomics: What Do We Know about the Genetics of Cancer in Domestic Cats? Vet Sci China 2022;9(10). https://doi.org/10.3390/vetsci9100547.
46. Sutter NB, Ostrander EA. Dog star rising: the canine genetic system. Nat Rev Genet 2004;5(12):900–10.
47. Boyko AR, Quignon P, Li L, et al. A simple genetic architecture underlies morphological variation in dogs. PLoS Biol 2010;8(8):e1000451.
48. Lloyd KCK, Khanna C, Hendricks W, et al. Precision medicine: an opportunity for a paradigm shift in veterinary medicine. J Am Vet Med Assoc 2016;248(1):45–8.
49. Katogiritis A, Khanna C. Towards the Delivery of Precision Veterinary Cancer Medicine. Vet Clin North Am Small Anim Pract 2019;49(5):809–18.
50. Garden OA, Volk SW, Mason NJ, et al. Companion animals in comparative oncology: One Medicine in action. Vet J 2018;240:6–13.
51. LeBlanc AK, Mazcko CN. Improving human cancer therapy through the evaluation of pet dogs. Nat Rev Cancer 2020;20(12):727–42.
52. Aupperle-Lellbach H, Grassinger J, Hohloch C, et al. Diagnostic value of the BRAF variant V595E in urine samples, smears and biopsies from canine transitional cell carcinoma. Tierarztl Prax Ausg K Kleintiere Heimtiere 2018;46(5):289–95.
53. Naka N, Ohsawa M, Tomita Y, et al. Prognostic factors in angiosarcoma: a multivariate analysis of 55 cases. Journal of surgical. 1996. https://onlinelibrary.wiley.com/doi/abs/10.1002/(SICI)1096-9098(199603)61:3%3C170::AID-JSO2%3E3.0.CO;2-8.
54. Wang G, Wu M, Durham AC, et al. Molecular subtypes in canine hemangiosarcoma reveal similarities with human angiosarcoma. PLoS One 2020;15(3):e0229728.
55. Wang G, Wu M, Durham AC, et al. Canine Oncopanel: A capture-based, NGS platform for evaluating the mutational landscape and detecting putative driver mutations in canine cancers. Vet Comp Oncol 2022;20(1):91–101.

56. Jahr S, Hentze H, Englisch S, et al. DNA fragments in the blood plasma of cancer patients: quantitations and evidence for their origin from apoptotic and necrotic cells. Cancer Res 2001;61(4):1659–65.

57. Schaefer DMW, Forman MA, Kisseberth WC, et al. Quantification of plasma DNA as a prognostic indicator in canine lymphoid neoplasia. Vet Comp Oncol 2007; 5(3):145–55.

58. Tagawa M, Shimbo G, Inokuma H, et al. Quantification of plasma cell-free DNA levels in dogs with various tumors. J Vet Diagn Invest 2019;31(6):836–43.

59. Kim J, Bae H, Ahn S, et al. Cell-Free DNA as a Diagnostic and Prognostic Biomarker in Dogs With Tumors. Front Vet Sci 2021;8:735682.

60. Prouteau A, Denis JA, De Fornel P, et al. Circulating tumor DNA is detectable in canine histiocytic sarcoma, oral malignant melanoma, and multicentric lymphoma. Sci Rep 2021;11(1):877.

61. Flory A, Kruglyak KM, Tynan JA, et al. Clinical validation of a next-generation sequencing-based multi-cancer early detection "liquid biopsy" blood test in over 1,000 dogs using an independent testing set: The CANcer Detection in Dogs (CANDiD) study. PLoS One 2022;17(4):e0266623.

62. Tagawa M, Aoki M. Clinical utility of liquid biopsy in canine oral malignant melanoma using cell-free DNA. Front Vet Sci 2023;10. https://doi.org/10.3389/fvets. 2023.1182093.

63. Wilson-Robles HM, Bygott T, Kelly TK, et al. Evaluation of plasma nucleosome concentrations in dogs with a variety of common cancers and in healthy dogs. BMC Vet Res 2022;18(1):329.

64. Caputo V, Ciardiello F, Corte CMD, et al. Diagnostic value of liquid biopsy in the era of precision medicine: 10 years of clinical evidence in cancer. Explor Target Antitumor Ther 2023;4(1):102–38.

65. Castro-Giner F, Gkountela S, Donato C, et al. Cancer Diagnosis Using a Liquid Biopsy: Challenges and Expectations. Diagnostics 2018;8(2). https://doi.org/10. 3390/diagnostics8020031.

66. Mathur S, Sutton J. Personalized medicine could transform healthcare. Biomed Rep 2017;7(1):3–5.

67. Manzari MT, Shamay Y, Kiguchi H, et al. Targeted drug delivery strategies for precision medicines. Nat Rev Mater 2021;6(4):351–70.

68. Wanebo HJ, Argiris A, Bergsland E, et al. Targeting growth factors and angiogenesis; using small molecules in malignancy. Cancer Metastasis Rev 2006; 25(2):279–92.

69. Normanno N, Gullick WJ. Epidermal growth factor receptor tyrosine kinase inhibitors and bone metastases: different mechanisms of action for a novel therapeutic application? Endocr Relat Cancer 2006;13(1):3–6.

70. London CA. Tyrosine kinase inhibitors in veterinary medicine. Top Companion Anim Med 2009;24(3):106–12.

71. Hahn KA, Ogilvie G, Rusk T, et al. Masitinib is safe and effective for the treatment of canine mast cell tumors. J Vet Intern Med 2008;22(6):1301–9.

72. Joo WD, Visintin I, Mor G. Targeted cancer therapy–are the days of systemic chemotherapy numbered? Maturitas 2013;76(4):308–14.

73. Imai K, Takaoka A. Comparing antibody and small-molecule therapies for cancer. Nat Rev Cancer 2006;6(9):714–27.

74. Rue SM, Eckelman BP, Efe JA, et al. Identification of a candidate therapeutic antibody for treatment of canine B-cell lymphoma. Vet Immunol Immunopathol 2015;164(3–4):148–59.

75. Maekawa N, Konnai S, Ikebuchi R, et al. Expression of PD-L1 on canine tumor cells and enhancement of IFN-γ production from tumor-infiltrating cells by PD-L1 blockade. PLoS One 2014;9(6):e98415.

76. Kumar SR, Kim DY, Henry CJ, et al. Programmed death ligand 1 is expressed in canine B cell lymphoma and downregulated by MEK inhibitors. Vet Comp Oncol 2017;15(4):1527–36.

77. Coy J, Caldwell A, Chow L, et al. PD-1 expression by canine T cells and functional effects of PD-1 blockade. Vet Comp Oncol 2017;15(4):1487–502.

78. Choi JW, Withers SS, Chang H, et al. Development of canine PD-1/PD-L1 specific monoclonal antibodies and amplification of canine T cell function. PLoS One 2020;15(7):e0235518.

79. Igase M, Nemoto Y, Itamoto K, et al. A pilot clinical study of the therapeutic antibody against canine PD-1 for advanced spontaneous cancers in dogs. Sci Rep 2020;10(1):18311.

80. Maekawa N, Konnai S, Nishimura M, et al. PD-L1 immunohistochemistry for canine cancers and clinical benefit of anti-PD-L1 antibody in dogs with pulmonary metastatic oral malignant melanoma. npj Precis Oncol 2021;5(1):10.

81. Minoli L, Licenziato L, Kocikowski M, et al. Development of Monoclonal Antibodies Targeting Canine PD-L1 and PD-1 and Their Clinical Relevance in Canine Apocrine Gland Anal Sac Adenocarcinoma. Cancers 2022;14(24). https://doi.org/10.3390/cancers14246188.

82. Whilde J, Martindale MQ, Duffy DJ. Precision wildlife medicine: applications of the human-centred precision medicine revolution to species conservation. Glob Chang Biol 2017;23(5):1792–805.

83. Sakthikumar S, Facista S, Whitley D, et al. Standing in the canine precision medicine knowledge gap: Improving annotation of canine cancer genomic biomarkers through systematic comparative analysis of human cancer mutations in COSMIC. Vet Comp Oncol 2023. https://doi.org/10.1111/vco.12911.

84. Chon E, Wang G, Whitley D, et al. Genomic tumor analysis provides clinical guidance for the management of diagnostically challenging cancers in dogs. J Am Vet Med Assoc 2023;261(5):668–77.

85. Chon E, Sakthikumar S, Tang M, et al. Novel genomic prognostic biomarkers for dogs with cancer. J Vet Intern Med 2023;37(6):2410–21.

86. O'Kell AL, Lytle KM, Cohen TA, et al. Clinical experience with next-generation sequencing-based liquid biopsy testing for cancer detection in dogs: a review of 1,500 consecutive clinical cases. J Am Vet Med Assoc 2023;261(6):827–36.

87. Rafalko JM, Kruglyak KM, McCleary-Wheeler AL, et al. Age at cancer diagnosis by breed, weight, sex, and cancer type in a cohort of more than 3,000 dogs: Determining the optimal age to initiate cancer screening in canine patients. PLoS One 2023;18(2):e0280795.

88. Ramón Y, Cajal S, Sesé M, et al. Clinical implications of intratumor heterogeneity: challenges and opportunities. J Mol Med 2020;98(2):161–77.

89. Sung JY, Shin HT, Sohn KA, et al. Assessment of intratumoral heterogeneity with mutations and gene expression profiles. PLoS One 2019;14(7):e0219682.

90. Sutherland KD, Visvader JE. Cellular Mechanisms Underlying Intertumoral Heterogeneity. Trends Cancer Res 2015;1(1):15–23.

91. Xalkori® (Crizotinib); Pharmacology Review. Center for Drug Evaluation and Research, U.S. Food and Drug Administration, NDA 202570, 2011.

92. Sprycel® (Dasatinib); European Medicines Agency, European public assessment report (EPAR) Scientific Discussion, 2006.

93. Davis, Hofmann NE, Li G, et al. A case study of personalized therapy for osteosarcoma. Pediatr Blood Cancer 2013;60(8):1313–9.

94. Imbruvica® (Ibrutinib); Pharmacology Review. Center for Drug Evaluation and Research, U.S. Food and Drug Administration, NDA 205552 (capsule), February 2014.

95. Honigberg, Smith AM, Sirisawad M, et al. The Bruton tyrosine kinase inhibitor PCI-32765 blocks B-cell activation and is efficacious in models of autoimmune disease and B-cell malignancy. Proc Natl Acad Sci U S A 2010;107(29): 13075–80.

96. Gleevec® (Imatinib); Pharmacology Review. Center for Drug Evaluation and Research, U.S. Food and Drug Administration, NDA 021335 (capsule),2001.

97. Tykerb® (Lapatinib); Pharmacology Review. Center for Drug Evaluation and Research, U.S. Food and Drug Administration, NDA 022059, 2007.

98. Lynparza® (Olaparib); Pharmacology Review. Center for Drug Evaluation and Research, U.S. Food and Drug Administration, NDA 206162 (capsule), 2014.

99. Ibrance® (Palbociclib); Pharmacology Review. Center for Drug Evaluation and Research, U.S. Food and Drug Administration, NDA 207103 (capsule), 2015.

100. Rapamune® (Sirolimus/Rapamycin); Pharmacology Review. Center for Drug Evaluation and Research, U.S. Food and Drug Administration, NDA 021083, 1999.

101. Nexavar® (Sorafenib); Pharmacology Review. Center for Drug Evaluation and Research, U.S. Food and Drug Administration, NDA 021923, 2005.

102. Mekinist® (Trametinib); Pharmacology Review. Center for Drug Evaluation and Research, U.S. Food and Drug Administration, NDA 204114, 2013.

103. Takada MMS, Jones A, Onsager A, et al. Phase I clinical trial to evaluate the tolerability of trametinib in dogs with cancer, In: Veterinary Cancer Society Annual Meeting, 2022; Norfolk, VA, 44.

104. Zolinza® (Vorinostat); Pharmacology Review. Center for Drug Evaluation and Research, U.S. Food and Drug Administration, NDA 021991, 2006.

Updates in Osteosarcoma

Jeffrey N. Bryan, DVM, MS, PhD

KEYWORDS

- Cancer • Osteosarcoma • Ablation • Radiopharmaceutical • Genomics
- PET imaging

KEY POINTS

- Pathologic evaluation of tumors with specific subtyping can improve prognostication for dogs with osteosarcoma (OSA).
- Limb-sparing accomplished by surgical as well as radiation techniques with chemotherapy yield long-term survival similar to that of amputation and chemotherapy.
- Multidimensional imaging including computed tomography (CT), PET/CT, and MRI can better characterize the extent of tumor and metastasis as well as patient risks including postradiation pathologic fracture.
- Immunotherapy has contributed to increased proportions of long-term survivors of OSA.

INTRODUCTION

Clinical care of osteosarcoma (OSA) in companion dogs has been relatively static during the past 20 years. The disease of OSA can be described as one of "life and limb." The limb pain associated with the primary tumors requires intervention to relieve the pain because oral pain medications are rarely sufficient to provide comfort. Amputation has been the mainstay of care because the surgery is relatively simple to perform, reliably relieves the pain of the primary tumor, and ensures that the limb will not become painful again in the future. Because of the comparative value of canine OSA to human disease, surgical limb-spare techniques were developed in the 1980s that continue to be used.[1,2] Radiation was identified in the 1990s as a source of palliation for OSA bone pain.[3] The primary threat to the life of a dog with OSA is metastatic disease with the vast majority (72%) dying of metastasis following amputation alone.[4] It has long been presumed that micrometastatic and microscopic disease develops early in the course of OSA, seeding the lungs and other organs with nests of cells that will prove deadly in the future. Supporting this, a recent necropsy study screened lungs of dogs euthanized for OSA without treatment looking for micrometastases.[1] A monoclonal antibody (TP-3) was able to detect micrometastases (5–50 cells) and microscopic metastases (>50 cells) in the lungs of 2 of 10 dogs

Comparative Oncology Radiobiology and Epigenetics Laboratory, University of Missouri Columbia, Ellis Fischel Cancer Center, 900 East Campus Drive, Columbia, MO 65211, USA
E-mail address: bryanjn@missouri.edu

examined. The authors observed that this was far less than the high number cases expected but nevertheless confirms the presence of microscopic disease in dogs with radiographically normal lungs.[1] Because of this high frequency of metastatic disease, platinum-based chemotherapy has been the standard of veterinary care following amputation or limb-spare to extend life.[5]

Although little has revolutionized care of dogs with OSA since the initial big advances of limb-spare and chemotherapy, new pathologic understanding, diagnostic modalities, and therapeutic advances offer hope for a future with longer survival. The era of massively parallel nucleic acid sequencing has laid bare the genomic and transcriptomic alterations that underlie the aggressive nature of OSA in dogs and humans. The increasing availability of computed tomography (CT), magnetic resonance imaging (MRI), and positron emission tomography (PET) are improving the assessment of the primary tumors and screening for metastatic disease that improve clinical decision-making in advance of therapeutic decisions. Improved surgical techniques, radiation delivery systems, and ablative technologies allow limb-sparing with both palliative and definitive intent for dogs unlikely to function well with only 3 legs. The current standard of carboplatin chemotherapy following amputation has been defined, and new approaches to chemotherapy design, immunotherapy application, and radiopharmaceutical treatment are opening horizons for future improvements in metastatic disease-free life and metastatic disease care. The hope and promise of these innovations is the advancement of care for all species as we innovate in our companion dogs. This review summarizes advances reported in the last 3 years in OSA in dogs.

DISEASE RISK, PATHOLOGY, AND GENETICS/GENOMICS

Breed predispositions toward the development of OSA have long been described. Recent study confirms that breed is a significant risk factor with the 4 highest risk breeds reported to be Scottish Deerhound, Leonberger, Great Dane, and Rottweiler.[6,7] Along with breed, dolichocephaly and large adult body size were identified as risk factors for OSA with chondrodysplasia and brachycephaly being associated with lower risk.[6] Body condition score has also been also positively associated with risk.[7] Such knowledge can direct novel screening technologies to at-risk individuals and possibly help lower the risk of breeds already at high risk through lifestyle management.

Pathology relies on light microscopy with immunohistochemistry to define tumor diagnoses and biological characteristics. Morphologic subtypes of OSA can have different clinical outcomes when properly categorized. Surface OSA (periosteal and parosteal) have been reported to have a better prognosis compared with medullary origin disease.[8] A pathology study dividing OSA samples into 3 subtypes found significantly longer mean survival in dogs with the fibroblastic morphology compared with the osteoblastic or chondroblastic morphology (546 days vs 257 or 170 days, respectively).[9] Immunohistochemical attempts to definitively separate these subtypes were not successful.[9] New technological and computing approaches are changing the way pathologic diagnoses are reached in some histologies. Unlocking the subtypes of OSA to predict clinical behavior has been challenging; recently, a convolutional neural network was applied to multiple features of 306 canine OSA samples from Comparative Oncology Trials Consortium (COTC) study subjects to subclassify them.[10] Three distinct clusters of response to standard therapy were uncovered,[10] suggesting that outcome prediction may be possible before therapy in the future.

Genomic descriptions of OSA are increasingly frequent, supporting the shared chromosomal, genetic, and epigenetic abnormalities between dog and human.[11–18]

Estimates of heritability and alterations in gene expression have been identified in high-risk breeds including the Rottweiler, Irish Wolfhound, and Leonberger.[12–14] Whole genome, transcriptome, and methylome sequencing have identified chromosomal rearrangements, gene mutations, alterations in gene expression, alterations in microRNA expression, and DNA methylation pattern changes similar to human cell line and tumor samples.[11,15–17,19] Silencing of the phosphatase and tensin homolog (PTEN) gene is important to human OSA, often by DNA methylation silencing.[20] Although epigenetic silencing was not observed in canine OSA samples, reduction in PTEN copy numbers was present in 23 of 95 samples.[20] Due to the syntenic rearrangement of the canine genome, the PTEN gene resides on distal chromosome 26, making it susceptible to homozygous deletion.[15,20] As more genomic data are generated elucidating drivers and pathways critical to OSA survival and metastasis, hope is high for new targeted therapies to extend the lives of these dogs.

IMAGING OSTEOSARCOMA

Multidimensional imaging in the form of CT, MRI, and PET/CT has become more frequently available to veterinary patients in the last decade. PET imaging can be used to stage dogs with cancer using fluorine-18-fluorodeoxyglucose (^{18}F-FDG). A retrospective study of 71 dogs with appendicular OSA evaluated the use of ^{18}F-FDG in staging patients before therapy decisions.[21] Comparing the radiopharmaceutical uptake, CT appearance, and contrast enhancement patterns, the radiologists identified 17 out of 71 dogs with a high suspicion and 12 out of 71 dogs with confirmation of metastatic OSA or second malignancy (8 out of 71 confirmed to have both).[21] This study confirmed the utility of ^{18}F-FDG PET imaging for staging of appendicular OSA. The same group evaluated ^{18}F-FDG PET for the detection of lymph node metastasis of OSA.[22] Retrospectively, maximum standard uptake values (SUV$_{max}$) of nodes determined to be metastatic by cytology or biopsy were compared with nodes that were not metastatic.[22] The metastatic nodes had statistically higher SUV$_{max}$ than the nonmetastatic node; further prospective analysis will be necessary to confirm the clinical utility of this observation.[22] The ^{18}F-FDG PET scan allows the measurement of metabolic tumor volume and total lesion glycolysis along with SUV$_{max}$, parameters used in human medicine to quantify tumor characteristics. In a retrospective analysis of the association of these parameters with survival, cutoff values could be defined that separated dogs into those more likely to survive greater than 1 year versus those surviving less than 1 year.[23] Comparing whole body CT to ^{18}F-FDG whole body PET/CT, the addition of the PET imaging improves sensitivity to metastatic and comorbid malignant lesions.[24] This retrospective finding supports the potential utility of such metabolic characterization in determining prognosis for dogs with OSA. In addition to ^{18}F-FDG, ^{18}F-labeled fluorothymidine (^{18}F-FLT) can be used to stage dogs with OSA (**Fig. 1**).

Axial OSA can be a particularly challenging location to manage for a long-term clinical benefit. Precise identification of location and margins is important to surgical or radiation decision-making to control the primary disease. Vertebral OSA is particularly debilitating when spinal cord compression develops. Identifying the disease early and accurately is important. MRI is frequently used in assessing spinal lesions for possible surgical decompression. MRI characteristics of malignancy include involvement of the vertebral body with hyperintense signal on T2, short tau inversion, T1, and T1-weighted gradient echo sequences.[25] Additionally, the presence of bone sclerosis was significantly associated with OSA over other malignancies.[25] For bony lesions of the cranium or vertebrae, signal heterogeneity on T2 sequences, contrast

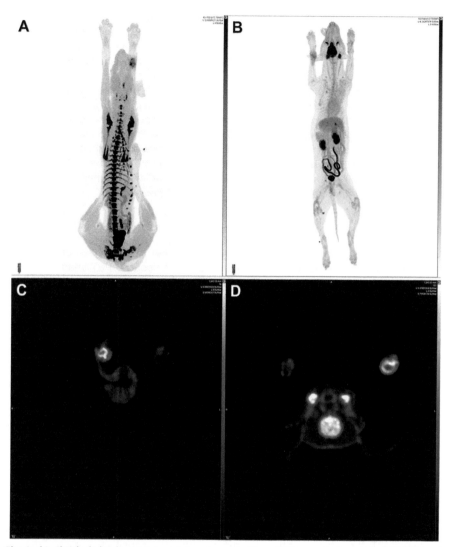

Fig. 1. (*A, B*) Whole body maximum intensity projections (MIP, panels *A* and *B*) of ^{18}F-FLT and ^{18}F-FDG, and (*C, D*) axial projections of ^{18}F-FLT and ^{18}F-FDG, PET images of 2 different dogs with OSA of the distal radius. Note that the ^{18}F-FLT is accumulated by mitotically active cells, highlighting the cycling bone marrow, areas of inflammation, as well as the tumor visible in the distal radius. The ^{18}F-FDG is accumulated by glucose-utilizing cells causing different distribution pattern from ^{18}F-FLT, highlighting the brain, salivary glands, gall bladder neck, kidneys, bladder, active intestines, active lymph nodes, as well as the tumor visible in the opposite distal radius.

enhancement, compression, and osteolysis should raise concern for OSA.[26] Thoracic body wall OSA location can be managed surgically if identified at a resectable size and before the development of gross metastatic disease. In a multi-institutional retrospective study of 58 cases of thoracic body wall tumors imaged by CT, 56 tumors were malignant sarcomas including chondrosarcomas (CSA), hemangiosarcomas (HSA), and OSA.[27] Dogs with OSA were statistically more likely to have a single rib involved than dogs with CSA.[27] Sternal lymphadenopathy was more likely to occur in dogs with OSA and HSA than dogs with CSA.[27] Features including pulmonary metastases and pleural effusion were not associated with one histology over others.[27] Mineral attenuation was also not helpful in distinguishing OSA from CSA.[27] Ultimately, biopsy of surgical specimens is necessary to distinguish among the common thoracic wall sarcomas.

SURGICAL AND RADIATION LIMB-SPARING THERAPY

Surgical limb-sparing procedures have radically changed functionality for human patients with OSA. Techniques now used in humans were shown to be feasible in companion dogs before their translation to the oncology clinic.[2] Although most limb-sparing surgeries require replacing the resected bone with an implant, procedures for OSA tumors of the ulna have the unique property of not requiring a weight-bearing solution. A retrospective study evaluated the outcome of radiation therapy, either stereotactic body radiotherapy or coarse-fractionated radiotherapy, or ulnectomy with or without chemotherapy for OSA in the ulna of dogs. Both forms of radiation therapy resulted in future pathologic fracture in a substantial proportion of cases (33.3% and 41.7%, respectively).[28] None of the dogs undergoing ulnectomy required further surgical stabilization or intervention.[28] Local recurrence of the tumors occurred in all groups.[28] Longest survival was associated with chemotherapy administration and ulnectomy in this series.[28] This study demonstrates the feasibility of simple ulnectomy to manage OSA in that bone.

Stereotactic body radiation therapy (SBRT) has been increasingly used for minimally invasive limb-sparing of appendicular OSA. A multi-institutional, retrospective study of 130 anatomic locations treated in 123 dogs assessed response and outcome.[29] Of 98 evaluable dogs, 82 had maximal improvement in lameness a median of 3 weeks after treatment.[29] Of evaluable dogs, pathologic fracture developed in 41% with 21% undergoing subsequent amputation.[29] Of the 123 dogs, 83 received adjuvant zoledronate, and 119 received adjuvant carboplatin.[29] Median time to first event was 143 days and median survival time (MST) was 233 days.[29] Dogs that were amputated had a longer MST (346 vs 202 days).[29] Pathologic limb fracture has been reported as a frequent complication following radiation therapy for OSA in many studies. A single-institution evaluation of 127 appendicular tumors in 122 dogs identified 50 fractures in the cohort following SBRT.[30] Of the sites treated, distal tibia (6 out of 9) and proximal femur (2 out of 3) were most likely to fracture (66.7%).[30] The distal radius was the most likely to develop a transverse fracture.[30] To attempt to predict likelihood of fracture for dogs intended to undergo SBRT for OSA lesions, a scoring system for CT images to assign grade has been created.[31] The CT grade was based on degree of lysis, length of identified full cortical lysis, subchondral bone lysis, and ratio of length of affected bone to normal bone.[31] Increasing grade was positively correlated with development of fracture.[31] Independently, subchondral lysis was associated with a 2.2-fold risk of fracture.[31] These results highlight the benefit of careful CT evaluation before radiation therapy to educate the client on risk of future pathologic fracture.

Hypofractionated radiation therapy (RT) has been used for pain palliation of OSA for decades. A recent retrospective study of 51 dogs receiving either hypofractionated RT or fine-fractionated RT identified a higher fracture rate for dogs in the fine-fractionated RT group (83% vs 30%).[32] This study described a subset of dogs receiving zoledronate along with hypofractionated RT (7 dogs), none of which experienced a pathologic fracture, raising the possibility that adjuvant zoledronate could reduce or prevent pathologic fracture in appendicular patients with OSA treated with RT.[32] A retrospective study of 165 dogs treated with hypofractionated RT evaluated the effects of adjuvant bisphosphonates and chemotherapy on survival outcome.[33] Neither bisphosphonate drug (pamidronate vs zoledronate) nor timing of the drug (concurrent or following RT) had measurable impact on the outcome.[33] Further, neither chemotherapy administration nor amputation following RT had a significant impact on survival of the dogs in this study.[33] A bi-institutional retrospective study compared outcome between dogs receiving either SBRT or hypofractionated RT followed by chemotherapy.[34] Pain at the beginning of treatment was evaluated as an independent variable. In the multivariable model, for dogs treated with both radiation and chemotherapy, low baseline pain score and high radiation dose were associated with statistically longer survival, supporting the benefit of definitive SBRT and chemotherapy over hypofractionated RT and chemotherapy for longer survival.[34] All approaches to managing the primary tumor with radiation carry a risk of pathologic fracture, raising the concern of limb pain to the forefront once again.

ABLATIVE THERAPIES

Ablative therapies aim to destroy the OSA tumor tissue in situ. In some cases, the intent is to destroy the tumors minimally invasively and avoid major surgery. Other approaches intend to cause immunogenic death of the tumor to enhance an antitumor immune response, killing metastatic sites with the primary. Multiple mechanisms of ablative tumor therapy exist.

One group has evaluated the feasibility of microwave ablation of pulmonary metastatic OSA. Two dogs were treated percutaneously to ablate pulmonary metastatic lesions. One dog experienced pneumothorax postprocedurally that resolved.[35] Both dogs tolerated the procedure well, demonstrating tolerability and technical feasibility.[35] The approach was extended to primary radial OSA lesions. Six dogs underwent microwave ablation.[36] Two power settings were tested to assess tolerability.[36] Tumor necrosis ranged from 30% to 90% (median 55%) as assessed by histopathology.[36] No complications were observed during or after the procedures, supporting safety and feasibility.[36] Larger studies will be needed to evaluate midterm efficacy.

Another group has studied histotripsy of OSA tumors (**Fig. 2**). The investigation began with a study of excised OSA tumors embedded in gelatin then with overlying tissue intact.[37] Using a 500-kHz transducer, bubble clouds were generated at the focus in each sample, consistent with effective ablation.[37] Ablative zones were confirmed by histopathology in all samples, confirming feasibility of the technology application.[37] The approach was extended to 5 dogs with OSA treated with the same transducer at 500 pulses resulting in clinically relevant ablation volumes and good tolerability.[38] Treatment dose was escalated to 1000 pulses in a series of 9 dogs resulting in larger ablation volumes.[39] CT following histotripsy demonstrated radiographic changes in 8 out of 9 dogs.[39] The group continues to study the application of histotripsy to OSA.

High-intensity focused ultrasound has also been reported as a means of ablation of a single OSA lesion but is used more commonly for soft-tissue tumors.[40]

CHEMOTHERAPY

A seminal prospective study was published through the COTC that evaluated standard of care (SOC; amputation with 4 doses of carboplatin) versus SOC plus sirolimus with DFI and overal survival (OS) the primary endpoints.[41] A total of 324 dogs were enrolled in the study and no statistical differences were observed in outcome.[41] The median survival of the SOC dogs was 282 days and the SOC plus sirolimus was

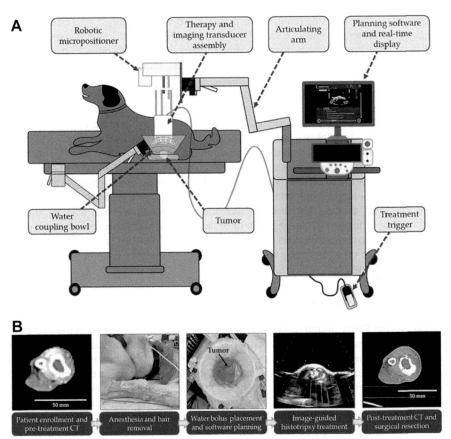

Fig. 2. (*A*) Experimental histotripsy setup. A robotic micropositioner was connected to an articulating arm to support the therapy and imaging transducers and submerged in a degassed water bowl coupled to the patient's tumor. (*B*) Study workflow. Patient-specific treatment plans were developing using pretreatment imaging assessments. Before treatment, patients were anesthetized, and the hair overlying the treatment area was removed. Automated histotripsy treatments were conducted using custom treatment planning software and monitored in real-time using ultrasound imaging. One day after treatment, post-treatment CT scans were collected before limb amputation. (Figure 2A was created with BioRender.com. Figure 2B. Ruger LN, Hay AN, Vickers ER, Coutermarsh-Ott SL, Gannon JM, Covell HS, Daniel GB, Laeseke PF, Ziemlewicz TJ, Kierski KR, et al. Characterizing the Ablative Effects of Histotripsy for Osteosarcoma: In Vivo Study in Dogs. Cancers. 2023; 15(3):741. https://doi.org/10.3390/cancers15030741.)

280 days.[41] It is worth noting that sirolimus trough levels were potentially low enough to abrogate beneficial effect.[41] This importantly established a well-documented prospective analysis of the outcome of amputation plus 4 doses of carboplatin.[41] Whether this should be the true SOC can be debated but the data set will serve as an important benchmark of outcome for amputation plus chemotherapy. Notably, carboplatin was administered between 10 and 21 days after surgery in this study.[41] A multi-institutional study evaluated the impact of amputation-chemotherapy initiation interval. Looking at a retrospective cohort of dogs, a significant difference in survival was identified between those dogs that received chemotherapy beginning 5 days or fewer after surgery

compared with those beginning more than 5 days after surgery.[41,42] The dogs that began chemotherapy within 5 days had a median OS of 445 days compared with the dogs that began chemotherapy after 5 days of only 239 days.[42] It should be considered that timing of chemotherapy initiation may be important to patient outcome.

Targeting chemotherapy to the tumor microenvironment might increase exposure of tumor cells to potentially lethal chemotherapy drugs. One such effort tested a novel bisphosphonate/doxorubicin conjugate (12b80) in 10 client-owned dogs in a dose-escalation study to evaluate safety.[43] Safety was established with no major adverse events or cardiac toxicity noted at a doxorubicin dose equivalent of 110 mg/m^2.[43] Dogs dosed at the highest level survived long enough to suggest a signal of efficacy.[43] A prospective study of zoledronate assessed the response of zoledronate as a single agent to control stage 3 metastatic OSA; 2 of 8 dogs experienced relatively short periods of stable disease and the disease-specific median survival was 92 days.[44] Further, 2 of 8 dogs experience grade III or higher adverse events including conjunctivitis, fever, hypocalcemia, and hyperphosphatemia.[44] Further advancements in targeted cytotoxic chemotherapy will be developed, and immunotherapy has become a reality for some dogs with OSA.

RECENT IMMUNOTHERAPIES FOR OSTEOSARCOMA

Since William Coley began studying the immune response to tumors in the late nineteenth century, science has pursued effective means of engaging the immune system and breaking tolerance to cancer cells to effect more cures of patients. Many strategies have been used since that time, and recent advances in human medicine with immune checkpoint inhibition have sparked broad enthusiasm for advancing cancer immunotherapy. Approaches as complex as engineered antibodies and chimeric antigen receptor T cells and as simple as small molecule combinations are being tested. The combination of high-dose losartan and toceranib has been shown to suppress OSA pulmonary metastatic disease.[45] Evaluation of the mechanism of action of the drug combination in these cases suggests that inhibition of the CCL2-CCR2 axis reduced monocyte migration and exerted a clinical benefit with an objective response in 25% of the dogs and stable disease more than 8 weeks in another 25%.[45]

One of the simplest forms of active immunotherapy is vaccination for tumor-associated antigens. One such approach has been a simple peptide vaccination against an extracellular epitope of the epidermal growth factor receptor (EGFR) that is often expressed on cancer. Investigators have identified increased titers against EGFR and HER2, CD8 T cell invasion of tumors, immunoglobulin G deposition on tumor cells, and even resolution of metastatic OSA lesions postvaccination.[46] The 12-month survival among the reported cohort of dogs receiving amputation, carboplatin chemotherapy (4–6 doses), and EGFR vaccine was 65% (95% CI 53%–75%).[46] This approach may be a relatively inexpensive and beneficial adjunct to the typical SOC therapy.

Bacterial-based cellular vaccines have been explored for cancer immunotherapy. A Salmonella-based vaccine was used to treat 20 dogs following amputation and 4 doses of carboplatin chemotherapy, beginning after the third dose.[47] Autologous or heterologous OSA cells infected with attenuated *Salmonella enterica* serovar typhi Ty21a were grown in culture and the supernatant harvested for dermal vaccination.[47] Compared with dogs previously treated with amputation and 4 to 6 doses of carboplatin, the vaccinates had a significantly longer time to metastasis (308 vs 240 days) and tumor-specific survival (621 vs 278 days).[47] Vaccinated dogs exhibited humoral responses as well as increased interferon gamma secretion on T cell stimulation with vaccine peptide.[47] A cryopreserved, attenuated transgenic Listeria vaccine containing the *HER2* gene was tested in addition to amputation and 4 doses of carboplatin chemotherapy.[48] Although survival data have not been published for this vaccine, the safety profile was unacceptable with 4 dogs culturing positive for the *Listeria* organism.[48]

Administration of a recombinant oncolytic vesicular stomatitis virus with added interferon beta and sodium iodide symporter genes (VSV-IFNβ-NIS) in the neoadjuvant setting followed by amputation and 6 doses of carboplatin proved to be tolerable and to induce changes in the tumor microenvironment that were distinct from the saline control patients.[49] A larger proportion of dogs treated with the VSV-IFNβ-NIS were long-term survivors compared with controls from the same institution as well as the COTC SOC patient cohort.[41,49] A chimeric human/dog vaccine against the chondroitin sulfate proteoglycan 4 retarded tumor growth in a murine model of OSA and was tolerable and generated antibody titers against the target antigen in companion dogs.[50] Some numerical increase in median survival was seen but was nonsignificant.[50] Conditionally replicative adenovirus bearing a CAV2 gene (OC-CAVE1) was injected into dogs following amputation or limb-sparing surgery.[51] Antibody titers against CAV2 were increased in all patients following virotherapy and some evaluations of cellular response to virotherapy were altered but no substantial increase in survival was noted.[51] These studies highlight the potential of "bugs as drugs" in increasing the immunogenicity of cancer cells, unmasking them, and breaking immune tolerance to the tumors.

In humans, checkpoint inhibition and agonists of activating molecules have revolutionized cancer immunotherapy. A flow cytometry evaluation of immune checkpoint molecules confirmed the presence of programmed death ligand 1 (PD-L1), member of the B7 immune checkpoint family (B7H3), and herpes virus entry mediator (HVEM) on the surface of OSA cells.[52] Immunohistochemistry studies of OSA lesions demonstrated the attendant lymphocytes to be confined to the periphery of the tumors with the core being an immune desert.[52] Immunotherapy strategies are aimed at breaking this immune tolerance and enhancing penetration of immune effectors into the tumor center. OX40 is a tumor necrosis factor receptor superfamily member that activates lymphocytes in an immune reaction.[53] Two canine-specific OX40 agonists were successful in activating canine peripheral blood mononuclear cells (PBMCs)suggesting the potential for upregulating an antitumor immune response in cancer-bearing dogs.[53] Similarly, interleukin-15 (IL-15) upregulates natural killer and T cell responses. Human recombinant IL-15 was evaluated in 21 dogs with pulmonary metastatic OSA delivered by inhalational route.[54] The study was designed to identify dose-limiting toxicoses (DLTs) and maximum tolerated dose (MTD) of the drug; secondary endpoints included progression-free survival and overall survival. The MTD was determined to be 50 µg administered twice daily for 14 days.[54] Of 18 evaluable dogs, 1 complete response and 1 partial response were noted; 5 dogs exhibited stable disease.[54] The approach is under further investigation.

Another approach to breaking tumor tolerance used a combination of an immunocytokine with immunomodulating radiation to induce antitumor immunity. Dogs with metastatic OSA received immunomodulating 2 Gy external beam radiation doses to their index tumor followed by an immunocytokine conjugate of an anti-GD2 monoclonal antibody (mAb) with IL-2 attached.[55] Because the disialoganglioside GD2 is frequently expressed on the surface of OSA cells, the delivery to the tumor microenvironment and localization of the IL-2 stimulation is facilitated by the mAb.[55] Dogs then received further treatment using a tumor microenvironment-targeted radiopharmaceutical (^{90}Y-NM600) to deliver at least 2 Gy to all of the metastatic lesions, thereby resetting the immunosuppressive microenvironment to break immune tolerance.[55] The approach was tolerable and is undergoing further study.

Cellular therapies are leading the way in human immunotherapy with the highest frequency of efficacy, particularly in lymphomas and leukemias. In 14 dogs with OSA, an activated T cell approach without chemotherapy was piloted using autologous vaccination harvested from the amputation specimen administered 3 times followed by apheresis and nonspecific activation and expansion of T cells.[56] The activated product was transfused into the dogs and they received low-dose IL-12 5 times following on an every-other-day basis.[56] From this cohort, the median disease-free interval (DFI) was 213 days and the overall survival was 415 days.[56] Five dogs survived beyond 2 years.[56]

Identifying patients likely to respond and monitoring the response of dogs undergoing immunotherapy will require new tools and biomarkers of disease and response. One technology that facilitates identification of subpopulations of cells with high sensitivity is single-cell sequencing. Recently, a group published an atlas of leukocytes of dogs affected by OSA compared with healthy controls.[57] A benefit of single-cell sequencing is the ability to identify subpopulations of cell types with greater sensitivity than flow cytometry. The primary difference in this study was that polymorphonuclear and monocytic myeloid-derived suppressor cell populations were increased in the dogs with OSA compared with healthy controls.[57] Myeloid-derived suppressor cells are known to protect the tumor from immune attack, and might be regulated in immunotherapy to break tumor tolerance. Monitoring circulating tumor cells (CTC) is another potential biomarker of disease and response. A group of dogs were followed after amputation, monitoring CTC levels in the blood. A spike in CTC number was observed in 12 of 15 dogs developing radiographic pulmonary metastases an average of 36.5 days before radiographic evidence of disease.[58] Dogs developing the CTC spike lived a shorter median time and had a 10-fold risk of death compared with those that did not.[58]

RADIOPHARMACEUTICALS

For decades, radiopharmaceuticals targeted to the bone to alleviate pain and target the tumor cells have been used in human and veterinary medicine. Early bone-targeted agents bound to the mineral matrix to deliver a palliative radioactive dose. Agents approved in humans for palliation (^{153}SM-EDTMP; Quatramet®) and therapy (^{223}RaCl; Xofigo®) bind to the hydroxyapatite in the bone, particularly where the surface is highly irregular in regions of tumors. Dogs with bone tumors have been treated with Samarium-153 ethylenediamine tetra(methylene phosphonic acid) (^{153}Sm-EDTMP) for both palliative and therapeutic effect.[59–61] A new generation radiopharmaceutical Samarium-153 (1,4,7,10-tetraazacyclododecane-1,4,7,10-tetramethylene phosphonic acid) (^{153}Sm-DOTMP) had some palliative effect on tumor pain and reduced ^{18}F-FDG intensity in the OSA tumor in some patients as well, suggesting possible therapeutic efficacy in the optimal application.[62]

A pretargeted strategy was recently published in which a bisphosphonate tagged with a click chemistry molecule was injected to localize to the bone followed by a chelated radioisotope also tagged with a complementary click molecule.[63] The study was the first to show that click chemistry will work successfully in a body that is near human-scale sized. The result is exciting because the pretargeting strategy would allow for short circulation of the radioactive portion of the drug even if the tumor-targeting vector had a long circulating half-life such as an antibody. The short radioactive circulation could optimize radioactive delivery to the tumor while minimizing exposure to at-risk organs.

Cell surface molecules have been targeted to deliver therapeutic radioisotopes to the cells. Insulin-like growth factor 2 receptor (IGF2R) expressed on OSA cells can be targeted in mouse xenografts of OSA with the antibody IF3.[64,65] Mice bearing canine OSA xenografts were treated with ^{177}Lu-IF3, suppressing tumor growth, demonstrating the therapeutic potential of the radiolabeled antibody.[66] The fully human IF3 antibody effectively targeted OSA tumors in companion dogs as demonstrated by Zirconium-89 PET/CT imaging.[67] Biodistribution of radiopharmaceuticals can be estimated using serial whole-body PET/CT imaging. Data from the biodistribution can then be used to calculate radiopharmaceutical dosimetry to tumors and target organs at risk. GD2 expressed on canine OSA cells was targeted using the human antibody hu3F8 labeled with Indium-111 (^{111}In).[68] Biodistribution measured by single photon emission tomorgraphy (SPECT)/CT showed uptake of the ^{111}In-hu3F8 in metastatic OSA lesions with favorable dosimetric calculations.[68] These 2 imaging studies show the feasibility of targeting OSA tumor cell surface molecules for targeted radioimmunotherapy. By targeting cell surface molecules rather than the bone matrix, each cancer cell might be targeted directly, homogenizing the radiation dose, eliminating the need for hydroxyapatite to be close enough to all tumor cells to deliver a therapeutically successful dose. Direct delivery to the cells makes feasible alpha-emitting radioisotopes whose deadly radioactive emissions travel relatively short distances in tissue. It is possible that in the near future more effective radioactive treatments will be available to companion dogs following these advances.

DISCUSSION

Canine OSA remains a prevalent disease and a daunting clinical challenge. Breed predisposition is strong with apparent genetically associated risk in the most common breeds. Continued work to identify markers of that risk for breeding decisions to lower risk is necessary. Genomic sequencing of OSA tumors is increasingly available; the further analysis of the enlarging data pool may yield diagnostic biomarkers for early detection as well as therapeutic targets for more effective personalization of therapy. In the meantime, routine pathologic subtyping of tumors to identify patients at higher and lower risk of early death may assist in stratifying therapy for more optimal outcomes.

Multidimensional imaging is clearly helpful in many aspects of decision-making for patient care. PET/CT with ^{18}F-FDG improves sensitivity for detecting metastatic lesions and second malignancies as well as offers potential prognostic value in quantitative analysis of radiopharmaceutical distribution. PET/CT offers improved performance over CT alone. CT allows assessment of bone structure to predict risk of pathologic fracture following SBRT and RT for pain palliation and limb-sparing. More routine systematic analysis of tumor CT images is advised to capitalize on the opportunity to select therapy that minimizes the patient's total risk of suffering. In spite of the advances in quality and resolution, CT, PET/CT, and MRI are not able to reliably distinguish OSA from other sarcomas, and biopsy remains necessary for definitive treatment planning.

Amputation remains the most expedient manner of relieving pain from primary OSA tumors and preventing its recurrence. Some dogs are not optimal candidates to be 3-legged, making limb-sparing options necessary. Surgery and radiation can accomplish this effectively and, with chemotherapy, deliver similar survival times as amputation. It may become evident over time that the potential immune stimulation of immunogenic cell death from radiation or ablative approaches or the inflammation resulting secondary to surgical site infection offer a reliable extension of life, especially when combined with immunotherapy such as immune checkpoint inhibitors. Until immune techniques are optimized, radiation and surgical limb-spare are effective means of controlling limb pain from the primary tumor.

Carboplatin has become the standard adjuvant chemotherapy for OSA. The outcome of the large prospective COTC trial was somewhat disappointing in that the 280-day MST was less than some earlier retrospective evaluation. The relatively short survival of roughly 9 months emphasizes the need for more effective targeting of micrometastatic disease in newly diagnosed patients. Targeted chemotherapies may offer improved efficacy in the future. Immunotherapy may prove effective in breaking immune tolerance and lead to more long-term survivals and cures in dogs with OSA. It is worth noting that to date, PD1 inhibition in human patients with OSA has not been extremely successful in providing large survival benefit or cure.[69] Nonetheless, data from past immunotherapy efforts provide hope and the novel approaches may be improved with time to benefit larger proportions of patients.

Radiopharmaceuticals have the potential to target tumor cells selectively and take advantage of applying lethal payloads to tumor cells while sparing normal tissue surrounding. These radioactive drugs have been used to target the immune microenvironment as well as the tumors themselves. Recent approvals of radioactive drugs for pancreatic and prostate cancers in humans give hope for similar drugs to benefit dogs and humans with OSA. Application will be limited by the regulatory requirements necessary to handle radioactive materials but the benefits may drive access for larger numbers of patients.

CLINICS CARE POINTS

- The Scottish Deerhound, Leonberger, Great Dane, and Rottweiler are predisposed to the development of OSA with apparent genetic associations.
- The fibroblastic subtype of OSA has a more favorable outcome than the osteoblastic or chondroblastic.
- ^{18}F-FDG PET/CT is more sensitive than whole body CT for metastatic and comorbid malignancy.
- SBRT with adjuvant chemotherapy can result in comparable survival to amputation and chemotherapy.
- Surgical ulnectomy can effectively manage a primary OSA lesion and, with adjuvant chemotherapy, result in prolonged survival.

DISCLOSURE

Dr J.N. Bryan serves on the scientific advisory board of ELIAS Animal Health who are the proprietors of an immunotherapy protocol described in this article. He receives honoraria when participating in advisory board meetings. He owns no stock or equity in the company. Dr Bryan received funding from ELIAS Animal Health to conduct a pilot study of autologous vaccination and activated T cell therapy in dogs with osteosarcoma. The results are published in the manuscript Flesner et al.[56]

REFERENCES

1. Kerboeuf M, Koppang EO, Haaland AH, et al. Early immunohistochemical detection of pulmonary micrometastases in dogs with osteosarcoma. Acta Vet Scand 2021;63(1):41.

2. LaRue SM, Withrow SJ, Powers BE, et al. Limb-sparing treatment for osteosarcoma in dogs. J Am Vet Med Assoc 1989;195(12):1734–44.

3. Heidner GL, Page RL, McEntee MC, et al. Treatment of canine appendicular osteosarcoma using cobalt 60 radiation and intraarterial cisplatin. J Vet Intern Med 1991;5(6):313–6.

4. Spodnick GJ, Berg J, Rand WM, et al. Prognosis for dogs with appendicular osteosarcoma treated by amputation alone: 162 cases (1978-1988). J Am Vet Med Assoc 1992;200(7):995–9.

5. Mauldin GN, Matus RE, Withrow SJ, et al. Canine osteosarcoma. Treatment by amputation versus amputation and adjuvant chemotherapy using doxorubicin and cisplatin. J Vet Intern Med 1988;2(4):177–80.

6. O'Neill DG, Edmunds GL, Urquhart-Gilmore J, et al. Dog breeds and conformations predisposed to osteosarcoma in the UK: a VetCompass study. Canine Med Genet 2023;10(1):8.

7. Williams K, Parker S, MacDonald-Dickinson V. Risk factors for appendicular osteosarcoma occurrence in large and giant breed dogs in western Canada. Can Vet J 2023;64(2):167–73.

8. Cook MR, Lorbach J, Husbands BD, et al. A retrospective analysis of 11 dogs with surface osteosarcoma. Vet Comp Oncol 2022;20(1):82–90.

9. Al-Khan AA, Nimmo JS, Day MJ, et al. Fibroblastic subtype has a favourable prognosis in appendicular osteosarcoma of dogs. J Comp Pathol 2020;176:133–44.

10. Patkar S, Beck J, Harmon S, et al. Deep domain adversarial learning for species-agnostic classification of histologic subtypes of osteosarcoma. Am J Pathol 2023;193(1):60–72.

11. Chu S, Skidmore ZL, Kunisaki J, et al. Unraveling the chaotic genomic landscape of primary and metastatic canine appendicular osteosarcoma with current sequencing technologies and bioinformatic approaches. PLoS One 2021;16(2):e0246443.

12. Letko A, Minor KM, Norton EM, et al. Genome-Wide Analyses for Osteosarcoma in Leonberger Dogs Reveal the Gene Locus as a Major Risk Locus. Genes 2021;12(12). https://doi.org/10.3390/genes12121964.

13. Momen M, Kohler NL, Binversie EE, et al. Heritability and genetic variance estimation of Osteosarcoma (OSA) in Irish Wolfhound, using deep pedigree information. Canine Med Genet 2021;8(1):9.

14. Simpson S, Dunning M, de Brot S, et al. Molecular characterisation of canine osteosarcoma in high risk breeds. Cancers 2020;12(9). https://doi.org/10.3390/cancers12092405.

15. Megquier K, Turner-Maier J, Morrill K, et al. The genomic landscape of canine osteosarcoma cell lines reveals conserved structural complexity and pathway alterations. PLoS One 2022;17(9):e0274383.

16. Mills LJ, Scott MC, Shah P, et al. Comparative analysis of genome-wide DNA methylation identifies patterns that associate with conserved transcriptional programs in osteosarcoma. Bone 2022;158:115716.

17. Das S, Idate R, Regan DP, et al. Immune pathways and TP53 missense mutations are associated with longer survival in canine osteosarcoma. Commun Biol 2021;4(1):1178.

18. Ayers J, Milner RJ, Cortés-Hinojosa G, et al. Novel application of single-cell next-generation sequencing for determination of intratumoral heterogeneity of canine osteosarcoma cell lines. J Vet Diagn Invest 2021;33(2):261–78.

19. Roth E, Ollenschlager G, Hamilton G, et al. Influence of two glutamine-containing dipeptides on growth of mammalian cells. In Vitro Cell Dev Biol 1988;24(7):696–8.

20. Sarver AL, Mills LJ, Makielski KM, et al. Distinct mechanisms of PTEN inactivation in dogs and humans highlight convergent molecular events that drive cell division in the pathogenesis of osteosarcoma. Cancer Genet 2023;276-277:1–11.

21. Crooks C, Randall E, Griffin L. The use of fluorine-18-fluorodeoxyglucose-positron emission tomography/computed tomography as an effective method for staging in dogs with primary appendicular osteosarcoma. Vet Radiol Ultrasound 2021; 62(3):350–9.

22. Slinkard PT, Randall EK, Griffin LR. Retrospective analysis of use of fluorine-18 fluorodeoxyglucose-positron emission tomography/computed tomography (F-FDG PET/CT) for detection of metastatic lymph nodes in dogs diagnosed with appendicular osteosarcoma. Can J Vet Res 2021;85(2):131–6.

23. Griffin LR, Brody A, Lee BI. The prognostic significance of metabolic tumour volume and total lesion glycolysis for dogs staged for appendicular osteosarcoma with fluorine-18 fluorodeoxyglucose positron emission tomography/computed tomography. Vet Comp Oncol 2022;20(1):59–68.

24. Brody A, Crooks JC, French JM, et al. Staging canine patients with appendicular osteosarcoma utilizing fluorine-18 fluorodeoxyglucose positron emission tomography/computed tomography compared to whole body computed tomography. Vet Comp Oncol 2022;20(3):541–50.

25. Hanot EM, Cherubini GB, Marçal VC, et al. MRI Features of Solitary Vertebral Masses in Dogs: 20 Cases (2010-2019). J Am Anim Hosp Assoc 2021;57(4): 189–98.

26. Tam C, Hecht S, Mai W, et al. Cranial and vertebral osteosarcoma commonly has T2 signal heterogeneity, contrast enhancement, and osteolysis on MRI: A case series of 35 dogs. Vet Radiol Ultrasound 2022;63(5):552–62.

27. Cordella A, Stock E, Bertolini G, et al. CT features of primary bone neoplasia of the thoracic wall in dogs. Vet Radiol Ultrasound 2023;64(4):605–14.

28. Griffin MA, Martin TW, Thamm DH, et al. Partial ulnar ostectomy, stereotactic body radiation therapy, and palliative radiation therapy as local limb sparing treatment modalities for ulnar tumors in dogs. Front Vet Sci 2023;10:1172139.

29. Martin TW, Griffin L, Custis J, et al. Outcome and prognosis for canine appendicular osteosarcoma treated with stereotactic body radiation therapy in 123 dogs. Vet Comp Oncol 2021;19(2):284–94.

30. Altwal J, Martin TW, Thamm DH, et al. Configuration of pathologic fractures in dogs with osteosarcoma following stereotactic body radiation therapy: a retrospective analysis. Vet Comp Oncol 2023;21(1):131–7.

31. Martin TW, LaRue SM, Griffin L. CT characteristics and proposed scoring scheme are predictive of pathologic fracture in dogs with appendicular osteosarcoma treated with stereotactic body radiation therapy. Vet Radiol Ultrasound 2022; 63(1):82–90.

32. Norquest CJ, Maitz CA, Keys DA, et al. Fracture rate and time to fracture in dogs with appendicular osteosarcoma receiving finely fractionated compared to coarsely fractionated radiation therapy: A single institution study. Vet Med Sci 2022;8(3):1013–24.

33. Ringdahl-Mayland B, Thamm DH, Martin TW. Retrospective evaluation of outcome in dogs with appendicular osteosarcoma following hypofractionated palliative radiation therapy with or without bisphosphonates: 165 cases (2010-2019). Front Vet Sci 2022;9:892297.

34. Nolan MW, Green NA, DiVito EM, et al. Impact of radiation dose and pre-treatment pain levels on survival in dogs undergoing radiotherapy with or without chemotherapy for presumed extremity osteosarcoma. Vet Comp Oncol 2020; 18(4):538–47.

35. Dornbusch JA, Wavreille VA, Dent B, et al. Percutaneous microwave ablation of solitary presumptive pulmonary metastases in two dogs with appendicular osteosarcoma. Vet Surg 2020;49(6):1174–82.

36. Salyer SA, Wavreille VA, Fenger JM, et al. Evaluation of microwave ablation for local treatment of dogs with distal radial osteosarcoma: A pilot study. Vet Surg 2020;49(7):1396–405.

37. Arnold L, Hendricks-Wenger A, Coutermarsh-Ott S, et al. Histotripsy ablation of bone tumors: feasibility study in excised canine osteosarcoma tumors. Ultrasound Med Biol 2021;47(12):3435–46.

38. Elorriaga MÁ, Neyro JL, Mieza J, et al. Biomarkers in ovarian pathology: from screening to diagnosis. review of the literature. J Pers Med 2021;11(11):1115.

39. Ruger LN, Hay AN, Vickers ER, et al. Characterizing the Ablative Effects of Histotripsy for Osteosarcoma: In Vivo Study in Dogs. Cancers (Basel) 2023; 15(3):741.

40. Carroll J, Coutermarsh-Ott S, Klahn SL, et al. High intensity focused ultrasound for the treatment of solid tumors: a pilot study in canine cancer patients. Int J Hyperthermia 2022;39(1):855–64.

41. LeBlanc AK, Mazcko CN, Cherukuri A, et al. Adjuvant sirolimus does not improve outcome in pet dogs receiving standard-of-care therapy for appendicular osteosarcoma: a prospective, randomized trial of 324 dogs. Clin Cancer Res 2021; 27(11):3005–16.

42. Marconato L, Buracco P, Polton GA, et al. Timing of adjuvant chemotherapy after limb amputation and effect on outcome in dogs with appendicular osteosarcoma without distant metastases. J Am Vet Med Assoc 2021;259(7):749–56.

43. Boyé P, David E, Serres F, et al. Phase I dose escalation study of 12b80 (hydroxybisphosphonate linked doxorubicin) in naturally occurring osteosarcoma. Oncotarget 2020;11(46):4281–92.

44. Smith AA, Lindley SES, Almond GT, et al. Evaluation of zoledronate for the treatment of canine stage III osteosarcoma: A phase II study. Vet Med Sci 2023;9(1): 59–67.

45. Regan DP, Chow L, Das S, et al. Losartan blocks osteosarcoma-elicited monocyte recruitment, and combined with the kinase inhibitor toceranib, exerts significant clinical benefit in canine metastatic osteosarcoma. Clin Cancer Res 2022; 28(4):662–76.

46. Doyle HA, Gee RJ, Masters TD, et al. Vaccine-induced ErbB (EGFR/HER2)-specific immunity in spontaneous canine cancer. Transl Oncol 2021;14(11):101205.

47. Marconato L, Melacarne A, Aralla M, et al. A target animal effectiveness study on adjuvant peptide-based vaccination in dogs with non-metastatic appendicular osteosarcoma undergoing amputation and chemotherapy. Cancers 2022;14(5): 1347.

48. Musser ML, Berger EP, Tripp CD, et al. Safety evaluation of the canine osteosarcoma vaccine, live Listeria vector. Vet Comp Oncol 2021;19(1):92–8.

49. Makielski KM, Sarver AL, Henson MS, et al. Oncolytic vesicular stomatitis virus is safe and provides a survival benefit for dogs with naturally occurring osteosarcoma. bioRxiv 2023;100736.

50. Tarone L, Giacobino D, Camerino M, et al. A chimeric human/dog-DNA vaccine against CSPG4 induces immunity with therapeutic potential in comparative pre-clinical models of osteosarcoma. Mol Ther 2023;31(8):2342–59.

51. Agarwal P, Gammon EA, Sandey M, et al. Evaluation of tumor immunity after administration of conditionally replicative adenoviral vector in canine osteosarcoma patients. Heliyon 2021;7(2):e06210.

52. Cascio MJ, Whitley EM, Sahay B, et al. Canine osteosarcoma checkpoint expression correlates with metastasis and T-cell infiltrate. Vet Immunol Immunopathol 2021;232:110169.

53. Ruiz D, Haynes C, Marable J, et al. Development of OX40 agonists for canine cancer immunotherapy. iScience 2022;25(10):105158.

54. Rebhun RB, York D, Cruz SM, et al. Inhaled recombinant human IL-15 in dogs with naturally occurring pulmonary metastases from osteosarcoma or melanoma: a phase 1 study of clinical activity and correlates of response. J Immunother Cancer 2022;10(6):e004493.

55. Magee K, Marsh IR, Turek MM, et al. Safety and feasibility of an in situ vaccination and immunomodulatory targeted radionuclide combination immuno-radiotherapy approach in a comparative (companion dog) setting. PLoS One 2021;16(8):e0255798.

56. Flesner BK, Wood GW, Gayheart-Walsten P, et al. Autologous cancer cell vaccination, adoptive T-cell transfer, and interleukin-2 administration results in long-term survival for companion dogs with osteosarcoma. J Vet Intern Med 2020;34(5):2056–67.

57. Ammons DT, Harris RA, Hopkins LS, et al. A single-cell RNA sequencing atlas of circulating leukocytes from healthy and osteosarcoma affected dogs. Front Immunol 2023;14:1162700.

58. Wright TF, Brisson BA, Belanger CR, et al. Quantification of circulating tumour cells over time in dogs with appendicular osteosarcoma. Vet Comp Oncol 2023;21(3):541–50.

59. Lattimer JC, Corwin LA Jr, Stapleton J, et al. Clinical and clinicopathologic response of canine bone tumor patients to treatment with samarium-153-EDTMP. J Nucl Med 1990;31(8):1316–25.

60. Barnard SM, Zuber RM, Moore AS. Samarium Sm 153 lexidronam for the palliative treatment of dogs with primary bone tumors: 35 cases (1999-2005). J Am Vet Med Assoc 2007;230(12):1877–81.

61. Vancil JM, Henry CJ, Milner RJ, et al. Use of samarium Sm 153 lexidronam for the treatment of dogs with primary tumors of the skull: 20 cases (1986-2006). J Am Vet Med Assoc 2012;240(11):1310–5.

62. Selting KA, Simon J, Lattimer JC, et al. Phase I evaluation of CycloSam (Sm-153-DOTMP) bone seeking radiopharmaceutical in dogs with spontaneous appendicular osteosarcoma. Vet Radiol Ultrasound 2023. https://doi.org/10.1111/vru.13274. Published online July 10.

63. Maitz CA, Delaney S, Cook BE, et al. Pretargeted PET of Osteodestructive Lesions in Dogs. Mol Pharm 2022;19(9):3153–62.

64. Prabaharan CB, Giri S, Allen KJH, et al. Comparative Molecular Characterization and Pharmacokinetics of IgG1-Fc and Engineered Fc Human Antibody Variants to Insulin-like Growth Factor 2 Receptor (IGF2R). Molecules 2023;28(15):5839.

65. Boisclair C, Dickinson R, Giri S, et al. Characterization of IGF2R Molecular Expression in Canine Osteosarcoma as Part of a Novel Comparative Oncology Approach. Int J Mol Sci 2023;24(3):1867.

66. Broqueza J, Prabaharan CB, Allen KJH, et al. Radioimmunotherapy Targeting IGF2R on Canine-Patient-Derived Osteosarcoma Tumors in Mice and Radiation Dosimetry in Canine and Pediatric Models. Pharmaceuticals 2021;15(1):10.
67. Allen KJH, Kwon O, Hutcheson MR, et al. Image-Based Dosimetry in Dogs and Cross-Reactivity with Human Tissues of IGF2R-Targeting Human Antibody. Pharmaceuticals 2023;16(7):979.
68. Fu Y, Yu J, Liatsou I, et al. Anti-GD2 antibody for radiopharmaceutical imaging of osteosarcoma. Eur J Nucl Med Mol Imaging 2022;49(13):4382–93.
69. Shi B, Chang J, Sun X, et al. A meta-analysis: the clinical value of PD-1 inhibitor or protein tyrosine kinase inhibitors in the treatment of advanced osteosarcoma. Front Oncol 2023;13:1148735.

Noninvasive Blood-Based Cancer Detection in Veterinary Medicine

Andi Flory, DVM, DACVIM (Oncology)[a,1,*],
Heather Wilson-Robles, DVM, DACVIM (Oncology)[b,c,d,1]

KEYWORDS

- Liquid biopsy • Cell-free DNA • Nucleosomes • Next-generation sequencing
- Cancer detection

KEY POINTS

- Noninvasive cancer detection using liquid biopsy techniques is becoming common place in both human and veterinary medicine.
- These tests often use blood-based analytes, such as proteins or cell-free DNA, to detect cancer.
- Although these tests can successfully detect many types of common cancers, not all cancers can be detected using blood-based tests.

INTRODUCTION

Cancer is commonly encountered in veterinary practice and has been reported to be the most common cause of death in adult dogs.[1] In 2020, it was estimated that there were between 83.7 and 88.9 million dogs in the United States and that 45% of households owned at least one dog.[2] Cancer represents a significant and widespread threat, given that approximately 1 in 4 dogs are expected to develop cancer at some point in their lifetime. Cancer risk increases with age,[3] affecting almost half of dogs aged older than 10 years.[4,5]

A cancer diagnosis not only represents a medical challenge to the veterinarian but also an emotional one. When dogs are in the senior stage of life,[5] deep bonds have often formed[6] between the owner and their pet, as well as the pet and the veterinary team that has cared for them. The impact of a cancer diagnosis is intensified in the

[a] PetDx, 9310 Athena Circle, Suite 230, La Jolla, CA 92037, USA; [b] Volition Veterinary Diagnostics Development, LLC 1489 West Warm Springs Road Suite 110, Henderson, NV 89014, USA; [c] Ethos Discovery, 10435 Sorrento Valley Road, San Diego, CA 92121, USA; [d] The Oncology Service, United Veterinary Health, 6651 Backlick Road, Springfield, VA 22150, USA
[1] Both authors contributed equally to this publication.
* Corresponding author.
E-mail address: aflory@petdx.com

Vet Clin Small Anim 54 (2024) 541–558
https://doi.org/10.1016/j.cvsm.2023.12.008
0195-5616/24/© 2023 Elsevier Inc. All rights reserved.
vetsmall.theclinics.com

senior dog-family unit, underscoring the need for an empathic and supportive approach to care.[6]

As preventative care continues to evolve for pets, they are living longer, making cancer a growing challenge in veterinary medicine. To face this obstacle and achieve the best outcomes for patients, early cancer detection is more critical than ever. Liquid biopsy tests offer some of the most promising tools to accomplish these goals. In veterinary medicine, early cancer detection has been conceptualized in 2 ways: early-*stage* detection (ie, detection of cancer at stages I or II) and early *clinical* (preclinical) detection (ie, detection of cancer before the development of clinical signs); both early-stage and early clinical detection have been associated with improved outcomes for a wide variety of cancer types in dogs.[7–20] With the new availability of simple, noninvasive blood-based cancer screening and detection tests, the hope is that more cancer cases may be detected earlier, providing more patient treatment options.

EARLY CANCER DETECTION IN HUMANS

Early cancer detection has well-established benefits in human medicine, which is why organizations such as the American Cancer Society[21] and the United States Preventive Service Task Force[22] have developed guidelines for the ages and frequencies to begin screening for common cancer types. According to the American Cancer Society, regular screenings starting at guideline-recommended ages can help diagnose cancer at an early stage, when treatment may be more successful or easier on the patient.[23]

In humans, early detection can save lives and improve outcomes for patients with many types of cancer.[24] The best example of this is colorectal cancer (CRC). Early detection has been associated with an almost 50% decrease in the mortality of patients diagnosed with CRC through screening tests.[25] This is likely due to the large differences in stage-dependent survival for patients with CRC where stage I patients have a 94% survival rate compared with only 11% in stage IV patients.[26] It is estimated that 63% of deaths due to CRC are due to a lack of screening, resulting in detection at later stages of disease.[27]

However, it should be acknowledged that the benefits of early detection are not universal across all cancer histologies. In humans, early detection has not been shown to improve survival for patients with thyroid, prostate, or breast cancer, even though early screening protocols are frequently implemented for these tumors.[28] In many cases, the tumors that are detected early are slow growing with long lead times. These tumors carry a favorable prognosis and likely would have a good outcome even if they were found by traditional means.[29] However, subsets within these populations benefit from enhanced screening, such as carriers of the germline mutations *BRCA1* and *BRCA2* for patients at risk of breast and ovarian cancer.[30]

Why do some patients benefit from screening while others do not? The answer likely lies in the biology of the underlying disease. In patients with low-grade early-stage breast cancer, these tumors are unlikely to develop into high-grade tumors over time. High-grade breast cancers have a different molecular signature than those that are lower grade, which are less invasive and have a lower metastatic potential.[31] This is not true for CRC. Nearly all stage IV CRCs started as an adenomatous or sessile polyp that ultimately progressed to a higher stage and more invasive carcinoma.[32] For this reason, early detection has been most successful in human cancers that have well-defined precursor stages with a high likelihood of malignant transformation over time.

Noninvasive techniques for early detection have been successfully applied in human oncology through several pathways. Screening of the general population through single cancer detection tests, such as Cologuard, have improved early detection of

CRC in people with no known family history or medical predisposition to this disease.[33] Although the sensitivity of this test for detecting CRC directly is low, the identification of a subset of patients benefiting from enhanced screening has led to improved outcomes and a decreased risk of mortality due to CRC.[33,34]

More recently, liquid biopsy tests for the purpose of multicancer early detection have become more commonplace in human medicine. A study by Liu and colleagues, published in 2020, demonstrated the utility of a multicancer detection and localization assay, which uses methylation signatures in cell-free DNA (cfDNA) to detect and identify the tissue of origin of cancers in the blood.[35,36] This study described a test that can detect more than 50 types of cancer, many of which do not have existing screening recommendations, with 93% accuracy. A follow-up publication using the same assay was the PATHFINDER study presented by Beer and colleagues in 2021.[37] In this study, for the first time, test results were returned to the clinicians for "real world" care pathway assessment using this tool. This study involved 6629 participants; 36 (0.5%) received a "Cancer Signal Detected" result when no evidence of cancer could be found during enhanced screening (false positive). Twenty-nine cases (0.4%) were considered true positive cases. Nearly half of the cancers detected in this group were early stage (stages I and II) and 71% of the cancers detected were cancer types with no current screening recommendations.[37] There was no diagnostic resolution for 27 patients (0.4%) at the time of data presentation. The sensitivity of this test for all cancers was just more than 50%, and sensitivity increased with stage (stage I: 16.8%, stage II: 40.4%, stage III:77.0%, and stage IV: 90.1%).[38]

Other liquid biopsy techniques have been used with success, leading to early detection and improved outcome in patients with gastric cancers, head and neck cancers, non-small cell lung carcinoma (NSCLC), breast cancer, CRC, pancreatic cancer, esophagus, liver, and ovarian cancer.[39–48] Additionally, liquid biopsy assays have been used to differentiate tumor grade or stage at diagnosis, providing clinically impactful information in a noninvasive way for patients with CRC, lung cancer, lymphoma (LSA), hepatocellular carcinoma, cholangio-carcinoma, chondrosarcoma, and Ewing sarcoma.[43,49–54] Although still controversial, early evidence suggests that liquid biopsy can, in certain cancers, provide a noninvasive method for early detection and improved outcomes.

EARLY CANCER DETECTION IN DOGS

Despite being the most common cause of death in dogs, there are currently no cancer screening guidelines in veterinary medicine. In the 2018 Life Stage Guidelines from the American Animal Hospital Association, preventive health-care recommendations for senior and geriatric dogs include physical examination and routine laboratory testing (complete blood count, comprehensive chemistry screen, and urinalysis) every 6 months and fecal testing for parasites, tick-borne disease testing, and heartworm testing at least annually.[5] However, regular wellness examinations in addition to the combination of tests recommended, while imperative for general preventive care, are unlikely to detect the majority of malignancies in asymptomatic patients. A recent study evaluating how cancer originally came to the attention of the veterinarian in more than 350 dogs demonstrated that most cases (88%) were detected due to clinical signs noted by the owner, meaning that patients were already symptomatic for their disease. In this study, only 4% of cancer cases were detected because of a wellness visit.[7] This underscores the need for novel tools and guidelines for the early detection of cancer.

One important factor in early cancer detection for canines is knowing when to start screening. A recent study examined the age at which cancer is typically diagnosed in dogs.[3] By reviewing data from more than 3400 dogs with cancer, it was determined that the median age at cancer diagnosis was 8.8 years; median ages at diagnosis were also reported by breed and based on weight.[3] The recommendation was to initiate screening 2 years before the median age at cancer diagnosis to increase the chance of early detection.[3,55] This means that all dogs should begin cancer screening by age 7; however, certain breeds and larger dogs, which were found to develop cancer earlier in life, should start screening at younger ages. For instance, the median age at cancer diagnosis was younger for Mastiffs, Saint Bernards, Great Danes, Bulldogs, Irish Wolfhounds, and Boxers (around 6 years of age). In these breeds, it may be prudent to initiate cancer screening earlier in life, at age 4. Knowing the typical age at cancer diagnosis for dogs of various breeds and weights can help veterinarians make more specific screening recommendations for individual patients.

The ability to detect cancer earlier is expected to result in tangible benefits for patients and their families. Earlier literature has shown improved patient outcomes with early stage and/or early clinical detection for a wide range of cancers in dogs, such as higher remission rates, longer remission durations, and longer survival times.[8,10–17,19,20] However, there may be other patient benefits as well, including decreased morbidity,[56–58] shorter hospitalization times,[58] and increased likelihood of being discharged from the hospital.[58] Additionally, there may be benefits for the family, such as having the time to pursue diagnostics and consider therapy, a wider array of treatment options to choose from, and a reduced need for medical management of cancer-specific clinical signs.[59] Finally, benefits for the veterinary care team may include the ability to schedule cancer surgeries allowing for planning and preparation rather than performing them on an emergency basis, having the time to pursue specialist consultation to help guide the family, and being able to offer an array of treatment choices.

Some of the most promising tools to help achieve the goal of early cancer detection in dogs are blood-based cancer detection tests—tests that involve the noninvasive sampling and analysis of biomarkers found in blood. The blood contains thousands of molecular components and often, only a small fraction is derived directly from cancer cells (**Fig. 1**).[60] Liquid biopsy techniques focus on the isolation of certain components for the detection of cancer to help establish a diagnosis or to help monitor the disease throughout the treatment process. These components may consist of circulating nucleic acids, circulating tumor cells (CTCs), tumor-specific proteins, nucleosomes, or extracellular vesicles (EVs) of all sizes.[24,61]

The past decade has seen the introduction of a variety of such tests to the veterinary field—from protein-based assays to genomic sequencing-based assays. Many of these tools are the subject of ongoing research, and several have already reached commercial availability in the United States. Broadly, these tests can be classified as quantitative or qualitative depending on how the analysis is performed, and protein-based or cfDNA-based depending on the biomarker being analyzed.

QUANTITATIVE APPROACHES TO BLOOD-BASED CANCER DETECTION

Most liquid biopsy assays involve the quantification of blood-based biomarkers for the assessment of cancer risk. The most common biomarkers used in quantitative-based cancer detection tests are proteins, although quantification of other biomarkers, including cfDNA, is also being studied.

Quantitative Assays

Protein-based assays are appealing because proteins are often stable for long periods of time and the assays are quick, require small amounts of biological sample, and are

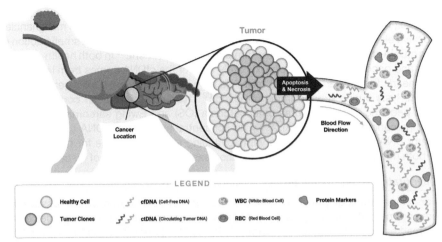

Fig. 1. Liquid biopsy involves the analysis of biomarkers in the blood. As cells die via apoptosis or necrosis, biomarkers are released into the bloodstream, including but not limited to proteins, extracellular vesicles, and fragmented DNA (referred to as "cell-free DNA" or "cfDNA"). If a tumor is present in the body, the subset of cfDNA fragments released from the tumor is referred to as "circulating tumor DNA" or "ctDNA." The identification of the presence of cancer biomarkers, such as genome alterations in ctDNA, or an increase in the quantity of tumor-associated proteins or cfDNA in a blood sample, indicates the likely presence of cancer in the body.

relatively easy and inexpensive. In humans, there are many protein-based cancer screening assays that are used frequently, including the prostate-specific antigen test, cancer antigen 125, carbohydrate antigen 15–3 (CA15 to 3), hepatocyte growth factor, lactate dehydrogenase (LDH), prolactin, tissue inhibitor of metalloproteinases 1, carcinoembryonic antigen (CEA), C-reactive protein (CRP), and thymidine kinase-1 (TK1) tests.[62–64]

Several of these protein biomarkers have also been investigated in dogs. CEA is a membrane glycoprotein associated with cellular adhesion. Elevated CEA concentrations have been found in the serum of intact female dogs with mammary tumors with a sensitivity 82.14% and a specificity of 95.24%.[65] The sensitivity of this enzyme-linked immunosorbent assay (ELISA)-based assay was increased to 100% for tumors larger than 3 cm.[65] CA15 to 3 is a transmembrane glycoprotein belonging to the *MUC-1* family that plays a role in immunosuppression and cancer cell dissemination during carcinogenesis. Elevated CA15 to 3 concentrations have also been associated with mammary tumors in intact female dogs.[66,67] LDH is an enzyme associated with the conversion of pyruvate to lactate and is often elevated at times of high metabolic demand, such as in cancer. Elevated serum LDH concentrations have been found in dogs with LSA and mammary tumors.[66,68]

Autoantibodies are proteins in the blood that target tumor associated antigens (TAAs). These autoantibodies have been found in the serum of patients at much higher concentrations than TAAs, especially in early-stage disease because the immune system will often amplify a clone and increase the expression of autoantibodies, even to a single TAA at low concentrations.[69] They are often found months to years before the cancer can be detected, depending on the rate of cancer progression.[70]

A final quantitative cancer screening assay that is being studied is based on the concentration of cfDNA in plasma. CfDNA concentrations have been found to be elevated in people and dogs with cancer.[44,71–75] A recent human study by Mattox and colleagues, reported that while oncology patients with a variety of epithelial malignancies do have elevations in cfDNA compared with healthy individuals, only a small fraction of this cfDNA is from tumor cells or the tumor microenvironment.[60] In both healthy individuals and oncology patients, approximately 70% of the cfDNA comes from leukocytes and nearly three-quarters of that cfDNA is from neutrophils, even after genomic DNA due to lysis during processing is removed.[62] This finding has been corroborated in both pediatric tumors such as osteosarcoma (OS) and Ewing sarcoma and in dogs with hemangiosarcoma (HSA).[76,77] The concentration of both cfDNA and circulating tumor DNA (ctDNA) do increase with advancing stage of disease for many cancers in both humans and dogs making detection easier at later stages of disease.[76–79]

Quantitative Assays Commercially Available for Dogs

For canine oncology patients, there are a few protein-based quantitative assays that are commercially available for the purposes of cancer screening. The first uses a dual biomarker algorithm combining serum CRP and TK1 concentrations to create a Cancer Risk Assessment (CRA) score. The specificity of an elevated CRA in a study of 360 apparently healthy dogs was 91% when CRP was elevated and 98% with CRP was very elevated. Additionally, a serum TK1 concentration greater than 30 U/L has been associated with a worse prognosis in dogs with lymphoma.[80]

Another commercially available cancer screening test for dogs and cats uses serum concentrations of onconeural autoantibodies to screen for cancer and other neurologic diseases. The company recommends using this test in animals with active neurologic signs and those cats and dogs predisposed to cancer. Although the company lists 21 cancers and 14 neurologic diseases that can be identified with this assay, no publications could be found describing the accuracy or utility of this test at the time of writing.

Detection of elevated plasma nucleosome concentrations is also commercially available as a cancer screening test for dogs. This assay uses an ELISA directed at histone 3.1 (H3.1) to quantify the concentration of intact nucleosomes in plasma. This test has been shown to identify up to 18 different histologic types of cancer but performs best for systemic cancers such as LSA, HSA, and histiocytic sarcoma.[81] When all cancers were considered, the sensitivity of this assay was 49.8% with a specificity of 97% and the area under the curve for the receiver operating characteristic curve was 68.7%.[81] The test was able to identify 82% of HSA cases and 74% of LSA cases with a specificity of 97%.[78,79] The test was also able to pick up two-thirds of patients with stage I disease for both LSA and HSA. For both HSA and LSA, plasma nucleosome concentrations increased with increasing stage of disease.[78,79]

Collectively, quantitative approaches to blood-based cancer detection may offer an affordable and accessible option for cancer screening in asymptomatic but high-risk patients. One important limitation to consider when using these tests is that a variety of noncancer conditions, such as sepsis, inflammation, trauma, surgery, and immune-mediated disease may confound the results because they can cause an elevation of the biomarker being measured.[72,82–87] For this reason, these tests are typically only recommended for asymptomatic, apparently healthy dogs when the test is being used as a cancer screening tool.

Additionally, depending on the assay, patient preparation (such as a requirement for fasting with the nucleosome-based test), blood collection practices, sample handling, and blood collection tube type can impact results and even cause false positives, so standardization and understanding of best practices to prevent spurious elevation of the biomarker being measured is paramount to developing a reliable and reproducible result.

QUALITATIVE APPROACH TO BLOOD-BASED CANCER DETECTION IN DOGS

An alternative blood-based cancer detection test in dogs takes a more qualitative approach to analysis and involves next-generation sequencing (NGS) to look for the presence of cancer-associated genomic alterations in cfDNA.[88] The presence of genomic alterations detected in plasma cfDNA were first reported in human patients with lung cancer[89] and human patients with head and neck cancer[90] in 1996, and in dogs in 2021.[91] This blood-based genomic profiling has been widely adopted in human medicine for multiple clinical uses, including for cancer screening, detection of molecular residual disease following therapy, and treatment response monitoring.[92] Additionally, the US Food and Drug Administration (FDA)-approved companion diagnostics exist for a variety of cancer types in people, including NSCLC, breast cancer, prostate cancer, and CRC.[90,93–97]

The underlying premise of NGS-based assays is that genomic alterations are the root cause of cancer, and detection of genomic alterations in cfDNA indicates the likely presence of cancer in the body. CfDNA can be extracted and analyzed using NGS to look for the presence of somatic alterations that originate from malignant tumor cells present in the body. This can include single nucleotide variants, insertions, deletions, copy number variants, and translocations.[90] A variety of approaches and methodologies can be used to detect genomic alterations via NGS-based assays, including targeted panels, whole exome sequencing, or whole genome sequencing.[98,99]

If a malignant tumor is present in the body, cancer cells release ctDNA that can represent DNA from multiple regions or metastatic sites in the body.[100] Indeed, studies in both people and dogs have demonstrated that the variety of genomic alterations present in a tumor (intratumor heterogeneity) or across tumors (intertumor heterogeneity) can be collectively in the blood, whereas this genomic heterogeneity may be missed when sampling individual sites within a patient's cancer.[90,101] This ability for a blood sample to provide a noninvasive method to confirm the presence of disease and to allow genomic analysis of metastatic or difficult to biopsy sites is a particular benefit in human oncology, wherein liquid biopsy can reduce the need for repeated biopsy of metastatic sites to confirm metastasis or sequence metastatic lesions.

There is currently one NGS-based cancer screening test commercially available for dogs. The validation of NGS-based testing was performed in a study involving more than 1000 dogs with and without cancer.[55] NGS-based liquid biopsy was able to detect 30 distinct cancer types at a sensitivity of 55% in the all-comers group, and 62% for 8 of the most common cancers seen clinically.[55] For 3 of the most aggressive canine cancers (LSA, HSA, and OS), the detection rate was 85%. The specificity of the test (98.5%) was established using a large cohort of presumably cancer-free dogs with a thorough history and physical examination by their enrolling veterinarian; importantly, these patients were not excluded due to chronic or acute medical conditions that are commonly encountered in daily practice, or common skin and subcutaneous tumors such as lipomas and sebaceous adenomas.[55]

A real-world clinical experience study of NGS-based liquid biopsy was published in 2023, examining 1500 consecutive samples. This study found that the performance of NGS-based testing in commercial samples (where cancer status was unknown at the time of testing) matched or exceeded the results reported in the clinical validation study.[102] Furthermore, the study found an almost 90% relative observed positive predictive value—that is, in patients receiving a *Cancer Signal Detected* result that then had a workup, cancer was found in 89% of patients using a standard workup in the practitioner's office—and an 88% relative observed negative predictive value.[102] In that study, veterinarians were primarily using NGS-based testing for cancer screening in asymptomatic patients (median age of 9 years) or as an aid in diagnosis when cancer was suspected (median age of 10 years).[102] A variety of cancer types were ultimately diagnosed in patients that had NGS-based testing performed for screening purposes, suggesting that the addition of liquid biopsy to routine wellness visits may help to expand the number and types of cancer that can be detected preclinically.[102]

NGS-based testing offers some advantages to quantitative testing approaches— most importantly, that it can be used in dogs with a variety of chronic and acute conditions because DNA abnormalities do not typically occur outside of cancer. For this same reason, the false-positive rate of NGS-based testing is very low (1.5%–2.5%).[55,102] Additionally, cancer signal origin (CSO) prediction is possible based on genomic features associated with specific cancers: for example, a CSO prediction for hematological malignancy can be made in certain cases, based on copy number gains or losses involving specific chromosomes[103,104] or the presence of somatic alterations in the patient's genomic DNA (isolated from white blood cells). A CSO prediction in these cases was found to have an accuracy of 92.7% for the prediction of hematological malignancy (lymphoma or leukemia).[55] The major limitations to NGS-based liquid biopsy testing is that the cost is higher than quantitative approaches, the volume of blood requirement is larger, and the turnaround time may be longer; additionally, specialized cfDNA-optimized blood collection tubes are required to collect the sample.

Regardless of whether a quantitative or a qualitative blood-based cancer detection test is used, it is important to note that not all cancers are detected by these tests. With nearly all of these assays, cancer detection is known to increase with extent of disease in the body as well as tumor size in people[38,39,44] and in dogs,[55,78–81] with detection rates for the most widespread disease reported as 83.9% in people for stage III-IV disease and 87.5% for disseminated/metastatic cancers greater than 5 cm in dogs, and 27.5% for stage I-II disease in people and 19.6% for localized/regional 5 cm or lesser in dogs.[38,55] Additionally, some cancers release less cfDNA into the blood and are therefore more difficult to detect than others, such as cancers of the central nervous system or urinary tract. Therefore, blood-based cancer detection tests should be viewed as a complementary approach to cancer screening or workup for cancer detection, along with currently used practices.

ALTERNATIVE APPROACHES TO BLOOD-BASED CANCER DETECTION IN DOGS

There are a few additional liquid biopsy approaches that have been studied in dogs but do not fit well into the categories above; these include CTCs and EVs.

CTCs have been used as biomarkers for cancer because they migrate through the blood during the metastatic cascade. These cells are very rare, as few as 1 of every 10^6 to 10^7 nucleated cells in the blood is a CTC. Because of their scarcity, highly sensitive assays are required to enrich for and identify these cells.[105] Although there is one FDA-approved CTC specific test in humans, there is no such commercial offering in the veterinary market.[105,106] Although not approved for veterinary use, this test has been studied in dogs and has shown a sensitivity of 44% for detecting metastatic canine mammary carcinoma; in the same study, those dogs with CTCs identified in blood had a worse prognosis.[107] Another recent study evaluating CTCs in dogs with OS followed 26 patients at the time of amputation and throughout treatment. A spike in CTC concentration was detected in 12 out of 15 with radiographic evidence of metastatic disease 36.5 days before detection of metastasis and was associated with a shorter median survival time.[108]

EVs are membrane structured microvesicles that are secreted by both healthy and cancer cells.[109] Tumor-associated EVs play a role in nearly all aspects of cancer development and progression. These microvesicles contain much higher amounts of protein transcripts than whole cells that can be measured in the blood.[109,110] EVs also contain cfDNA and RNA that can be used for liquid biopsy. Isolation of EVs from the serum can intensify the signal but requires special equipment or kits and can be cumbersome.

OTHER APPLICATIONS OF BLOOD-BASED CANCER DETECTION TESTS

In addition to their use for cancer screening, liquid biopsy approaches can also be used for monitoring of human and veterinary patients following a cancer diagnosis.

Residual Disease Detection

Qualitative liquid biopsy approaches can be used to detect the presence of molecular residual disease following surgery, also called residual disease detection.[88] The detection of ctDNA following curative intent surgery has been demonstrated to be prognostic for cancer recurrence in a variety of cancers in people.[111–116] In dogs, the detection of ctDNA in the blood after surgery can be prognostic: patients with genomic alterations remaining in blood after excision of gross disease had a 2-fold higher likelihood of clinical disease recurrence within 6 months, compared with patients with negative NGS results.[117]

Treatment Response Monitoring

In humans, biomarkers are commonly used to determine the response to therapy in NSCLC, breast cancer, CRC, bladder and prostate cancers, among others.[118–121] There are few such markers available in veterinary oncology. TK1 and CRP have been used to assess treatment response and predict survival in dogs with LSA.[122] In one study, the pretreatment serum TK1 and CRP levels were significantly higher than dogs in remission and dogs with elevated serum TK1 and CRP pretreatment had a significantly shorter median survival time than dogs with low TK1 and CRP concentrations before treatment.[123]

Circulating plasma nucleosomes (H3.1) have also been used to monitor treatment response in a variety of malignancies. Plasma H3.1 concentrations have also been shown to reflect treatment responses in humans with CRC, pancreatic cancer, and lung cancer and in dogs with a variety of carcinomas.[78,79,124–129] In dogs with LSA, plasma H3.1 concentrations were found to better predict treatment response than either CRP or TK1, and these increases often preceded clinical evidence of disease progression.[129,130] Additionally, dogs with plasma H3.1 concentrations greater than 67.4 ng/mL at diagnosis had a shorter progression free survival than those with lower concentrations.[129]

Liquid biopsy techniques using ctDNA have also been used for treatment response monitoring in humans and dogs.[88] Depletion of the ctDNA fraction in the blood is often an indication of complete response to therapy.[130,131] In many cases, ctDNA will increase in the serum before recurrence of the tumor is clinically evident.[131] Identification of patient-specific or disease-specific mutations can also be monitored in the blood providing a highly sensitive marker for disease progression or recurrence.

Recurrence Monitoring

Both quantitative and qualitative blood-based cancer detection tests are also available for recurrence monitoring. With quantitative-based tests, the patient is followed longitudinally with serial blood tests that compare the quantity of the biomarker over time. When significant elevations are noted, this can be an indication of cancer recurrence, even in the absence of clinical evidence of disease. For example, circulating H3.1 plasma concentrations have been used to monitor for disease recurrence. Elevations have been seen in cases with HSA up to 2 months before clinical evidence of progression was seen with computed tomography.[79] In a study of 37 dogs with lymphoma, plasma H3.1 concentrations were elevated an average of 18 days (range 6–80 days) before clinical progression was evident.[129]

In the case of the qualitative NGS-based test, serial blood samples are used to look for the reemergence of genomic alterations in blood, indicating "molecular recurrence" of disease.[132] An NGS-based test in dogs with a variety of cancer types was able to detect molecular recurrence before clinical recurrence in a subset of dogs with a median lead time of 168 days.[132]

Targeted Treatment Selection

Targeted treatment selection (aka personalized or precision medicine) involves the selection of therapeutics based on the genomic signature of an individual's cancer. Currently, targeted treatment selection is commercially available based on the genomic profile from testing tumor tissue directly, and blood-based approaches are expected to be available in the future. However, there are challenges to precision medicine approaches in dogs, including incomplete annotation of the canine genome (description of individual genes, identification of their protein or RNA product, and gene functions) and lack of complete knowledge of tumor context (mutations in specific cancers and their influence on cancer biology potentially influencing likelihood of precision medicine response).[133]

SUMMARY AND A LOOK TO THE FUTURE

The past decade has seen incredible advances in blood-based cancer detection in people and in dogs—yet this represents only a small glimpse of the benefits these tests can provide to patients. The clinical uses of this technology range from screening asymptomatic individuals for early detection to use as an aid in diagnosis when cancer is suspected, to cancer monitoring both during and after treatment. The coming years will likely see the addition of blood-based cancer detection to routine veterinary care, paving the way for enhanced understanding of the influence of early cancer detection, and allowing discovery of novel clinical factors related to prognostication, risk stratification, individualized treatment selection, therapeutic resistance, and enhanced patient management.

DISCLOSURE

Dr A. Flory is an employee and shareholder of PetDx. PetDx did not play a role in the study design, decision to publish, or preparation of this article. Dr H. Wilson-Robles is a paid consultant for Volition Veterinary Diagnostic Development (VVDD). VVDD did not play a role in the study design, decision to publish, or preparation of the article.

REFERENCES

1. Fleming JM, Creevy KE, Promislow DE. Mortality in north american dogs from 1984 to 2004: an investigation into age-size-and breed-related causes of death. J Vet Intern Med 2011;25(2):187–98.
2. Association AVM. Pet Ownership and Demographics Sourcebook Internet. American Veterinary Medical Association https://ebusiness.avma.org/files/ProductDownloads/eco-pet-demographic-report-22-low-res.pdf2022.

3. Rafalko JM, Kruglyak KM, McCleary-Wheeler AL, et al. Age at cancer diagnosis by breed, weight, sex, and cancer type in a cohort of more than 3,000 dogs: Determining the optimal age to initiate cancer screening in canine patients. PLoS One 2023;18(2):e0280795.

4. AVMA Cancer in Pets Internet. cited 2023 Aug 26. https://www.avma.org/resources/pet-owners/petcare/cancer-pets#:~:text=How%20common%20are%20neoplasia%20and ,rate%20of%20cancer%20in%20cats.

5. Creevy KE, Grady J, Little SE, et al. 2019 AAHA canine life stage guidelines. J Am Anim Hosp Assoc 2019;55(6):267–90.

6. Biller B, Berg J, Garrett L, et al. 2016 AAHA oncology guidelines for dogs and cats. J Am Anim Hosp Assoc 2016;52(4):181–204.

7. Flory A, McLennan L, Peet B, et al. Cancer detection in clinical practice and using blood-based liquid biopsy: A retrospective audit of over 350 dogs. J Vet Intern Med 2023;37(1):258–67.

8. Jagielski D, Lechowski R, Hoffmann-Jagielska M, et al. A retrospective study of the incidence and prognostic factors of multicentric lymphoma in dogs (1998-2000). J Vet Med A Physiol Pathol Clin Med 2002;49(8):419–24.

9. Treggiari E, Maddox TW, Gonçalves R, et al. Retrospective comparison of three-dimensional conformal radiation therapy vs. prednisolone alone in 30 cases of canine infratentorial brain tumors. Vet Radiol Ultrasound 2017;58(1):106–16.

10. Treggiari E, Borrego JF, Gramer I, et al. Retrospective comparison of first-line adjuvant anthracycline vs metronomic-based chemotherapy protocols in the treatment of stage I and II canine splenic haemangiosarcoma. Vet Comp Oncol 2020;18(1):43–51.

11. Treggiari E, Pellin MA, Romanelli G, et al. Tonsillar carcinoma in dogs: Treatment outcome and potential prognostic factors in 123 cases. J Vet Intern Med 2023; 37(1):247–57.

12. Spodnick GJ, Berg J, Rand WM, et al. Prognosis for dogs with appendicular osteosarcoma treated by amputation alone: 162 cases (1978-1988). J Am Vet Med Assoc 1992;200(7):995–9.

13. Rassnick KM, Goldkamp CE, Erb HN, et al. Evaluation of factors associated with survival in dogs with untreated nasal carcinomas: 139 cases (1993-2003). J Am Vet Med Assoc 2006;229(3):401–6.

14. Debreuque M, De Fornel P, David I, et al. Definitive-intent uniform megavoltage fractioned radiotherapy protocol for presumed canine intracranial gliomas: retrospective analysis of survival and prognostic factors in 38 cases (2013-2019). BMC Vet Res 2020;16(1):412.

15. McNiel EA, Ogilvie GK, Powers BE, et al. Evaluation of prognostic factors for dogs with primary lung tumors: 67 cases (1985-1992). J Am Vet Med Assoc 1997;211(11):1422–7.

16. Horta RS, Lavalle GE, Monteiro LN, et al. Assessment of canine mast cell tumor mortality risk based on clinical, histologic, immunohistochemical, and molecular features. Vet Pathol 2018;55(2):212–23.

17. Linden D, Liptak JM, Vinayak A, et al. Outcomes and prognostic variables associated with primary abdominal visceral soft tissue sarcomas in dogs: A Veterinary Society of Surgical Oncology retrospective study. Vet Comp Oncol 2019; 17(3):265–70.

18. Turek M, LaDue T, Looper J, et al. Multimodality treatment including ONCEPT for canine oral melanoma: A retrospective analysis of 131 dogs. Vet Radiol Ultrasound 2020;61(4):471–80.

19. Sorenmo KU, Rasotto R, Zappulli V, et al. Development, anatomy, histology, lymphatic drainage, clinical features, and cell differentiation markers of canine mammary gland neoplasms. Vet Pathol 2011;48(1):85–97.

20. Polton GA, Brearley MJ. Clinical stage, therapy, and prognosis in canine anal sac gland carcinoma. J Vet Intern Med 2007;21(2):274–80.

21. American Cancer Society Guidelines for the Early Detection of Cancer Internet. Available at: https://www.cancer.org/cancer/screening/american-cancer-society-guidelines-for-the-early-detection-of-cancer.html. Accessed July 16, 2023.

22. U.S. Preventive Services Task Force A and B Recommendations. Available at: https://www.uspreventiveservicestaskforce.org/uspstf/recommendation-topics/uspstf-a-and-b-recommendations. Accessed August 26, 2023.

23. Cancer.org Get Screened Internet. 2023. Available at: https://www.cancer.org/cancer/screening/get-screened.html HWR1.

24. Heitzer E, Perakis S, Geigl JB, et al. The potential of liquid biopsies for the early detection of cancer. npj Precis Oncol 2017;1(1):36.

25. Welch HG, Robertson DJ. Colorectal cancer on the decline–why screening can't explain it all. N Engl J Med 2016;374(17):1605–7.

26. Lansdorp-Vogelaar I, van Ballegooijen M, Zauber AG, et al. Effect of rising chemotherapy costs on the cost savings of colorectal cancer screening. J Natl Cancer Inst 2009;101(20):1412–22.

27. Meester RG, Doubeni CA, Lansdorp-Vogelaar I, et al. Colorectal cancer deaths attributable to nonuse of screening in the United States. Ann Epidemiol 2015; 25(3):208–13.e1.

28. Scudellari M. The science myths that will not die. Nature 2015;528(7582):322–5.

29. Lannin DR, Wang S. Are small breast cancers good because they are small or small because they are good? N Engl J Med 2017;376(23):2286–91.

30. D'Andrea E, Marzuillo C, De Vito C, et al. Which BRCA genetic testing programs are ready for implementation in health care? A systematic review of economic evaluations. Genet Med 2016;18(12):1171–80.

31. Schymik B, Buerger H, Krämer A, et al. Is there 'progression through grade' in ductal invasive breast cancer? Breast Cancer Res Treat 2012;135(3):693–703.

32. Choi Y, Sateia HF, Peairs KS, et al. Screening for colorectal cancer. Semin Oncol 2017;44(1):34–44.

33. Clebak KT, Nickolich S, Mendez-Miller M. Multitarget Stool DNA Testing (Cologuard) for Colorectal Cancer Screening. Am Fam Physician 2022;105(2): 198–200.

34. Stürzlinger H, Conrads-Frank A, Eisenmann A, et al, European Network for Health Technology Assessment EUnetHTA. Stool DNA testing for early detection of colorectal cancer: systematic review using the HTA Core Model. Ger Med Sci 2023;21:Doc06.

35. Liu MC, Oxnard GR, Klein EA, et al. Sensitive and specific multi-cancer detection and localization using methylation signatures in cell-free DNA. Ann Oncol 2020;31(6):745–59.

36. Taylor WC. Comment on 'Sensitive and specific multi-cancer detection and localization using methylation signatures in cell-free DNA' by M. C. Liu et al. Ann Oncol 2020;31(9):1266–7.

37. Beer T, McDonnell C, Nadauld L, et al, editors. Interim results of PATHFINDER, a clinical use study using methylation based multi-cancer early detection test. American Society of Clinical Oncology (ASCO); 2021. June 4-8, 2021; Virtual Meeting: J Clin Oncol.

38. Klein EA, Richards D, Cohn A, et al. Clinical validation of a targeted methylation-based multi-cancer early detection test using an independent validation set. Ann Oncol 2021;32(9):1167–77.

39. Guo X, Peng Y, Song Q, et al. A Liquid Biopsy Signature for the Early Detection of Gastric Cancer in Patients. Gastroenterology 2023;165(2):402–13.e13.

40. Mishra V, Singh A, Chen X, et al. Application of liquid biopsy as multi-functional biomarkers in head and neck cancer. Br J Cancer 2022;126(3):361–70.

41. Chang L, Li J, Zhang R. Liquid biopsy for early diagnosis of non-small cell lung carcinoma: recent research and detection technologies. Biochim Biophys Acta Rev Cancer 2022;1877(3):188729.

42. Alba-Bernal A, Lavado-Valenzuela R, Domínguez-Recio ME, et al. Challenges and achievements of liquid biopsy technologies employed in early breast cancer. EBioMedicine 2020;62:103100.

43. Zhou H, Zhu L, Song J, et al. Liquid biopsy at the frontier of detection, prognosis and progression monitoring in colorectal cancer. Mol Cancer 2022;21(1):86.

44. Phallen J, Sausen M, Adleff V, et al. Direct detection of early-stage cancers using circulating tumor DNA. Sci Transl Med 2017;9(403).

45. Church TR, Wandell M, Lofton-Day C, et al, PRESEPT Clinical Study Steering Committee, Investigators and Study Team. Prospective evaluation of methylated SEPT9 in plasma for detection of asymptomatic colorectal cancer. Gut 2014;63(2):317–25.

46. Watanabe F, Suzuki K, Noda H, et al. Liquid biopsy leads to a paradigm shift in the treatment of pancreatic cancer. World J Gastroenterol 2022;28(46):6478–96.

47. Herreros-Villanueva M, Bujanda L. Glypican-1 in exosomes as biomarker for early detection of pancreatic cancer. Ann Transl Med 2016;4(4):64.

48. Duffy MJ, Diamandis EP, Crown J. Circulating tumor DNA (ctDNA) as a pan-cancer screening test: is it finally on the horizon? Clin Chem Lab Med 2021;59(8):1353–61.

49. Gutteridge A, Rathbone VM, Gibbons R, et al. Digital PCR analysis of circulating tumor DNA: a biomarker for chondrosarcoma diagnosis, prognostication, and residual disease detection. Cancer Med 2017;6(10):2194–202.

50. Krumbholz M, Hellberg J, Steif B, et al. Genomic EWSR1 fusion sequence as highly sensitive and dynamic plasma tumor marker in ewing sarcoma. Clin Cancer Res 2016;22(17):4356–65.

51. Li M, Mi L, Wang C, et al. Clinical implications of circulating tumor DNA in predicting the outcome of diffuse large B cell lymphoma patients receiving first-line therapy. BMC Med 2022;20(1):369.

52. Li P, Liu S, Du L, et al. Liquid biopsies based on DNA methylation as biomarkers for the detection and prognosis of lung cancer. Clin Epigenetics 2022;14(1):118.

53. Chen VL, Xu D, Wicha MS, et al. Utility of liquid biopsy analysis in detection of hepatocellular carcinoma, determination of prognosis, and disease monitoring: a systematic review. Clin Gastroenterol Hepatol 2020;18(13):2879–902.e9.

54. Lapitz A, Azkargorta M, Milkiewicz P, et al. Liquid biopsy-based protein biomarkers for risk prediction, early diagnosis, and prognostication of cholangiocarcinoma. J Hepatol 2023;79(1):93–108.

55. Flory A, Kruglyak KM, Tynan JA, et al. Clinical validation of a next-generation sequencing-based multi-cancer early detection "liquid biopsy" blood test in over 1,000 dogs using an independent testing set: The CANcer Detection in Dogs (CANDiD) study. PLoS One 2022;17(4):e0266623.

56. Davies O, Taylor AJ. Refining the "double two-thirds" rule: Genotype-based breed grouping and clinical presentation help predict the diagnosis of canine splenic mass lesions in 288 dogs. Vet Comp Oncol 2020;18(4):548–58.
57. Marino DJ, Matthiesen DT, Fox PR, et al. Ventricular arrhythmias in dogs undergoing splenectomy: a prospective study. Vet Surg 1994;23(2):101–6.
58. Lynch AM, O'Toole TE, Respess M. Transfusion practices for treatment of dogs hospitalized following trauma: 125 cases (2008-2013). J Am Vet Med Assoc 2015;247(6):643–9.
59. Herold LV, Devey JJ, Kirby R, et al. Clinical evaluation and management of hemoperitoneum in dogs. J Vet Emerg Crit Care 2008;18(1):40–53.
60. Mattox AK, Douville C, Wang Y, et al. The origin of highly elevated cell-free DNA in healthy individuals and patients with pancreatic, colorectal, lung, or ovarian cancer. Cancer Discov 2023;13(10):2166–79.
61. Palanca-Ballester C, Rodriguez-Casanova A, Torres S, et al. Cancer epigenetic biomarkers in liquid biopsy for high incidence malignancies. Cancers 2021;13(12).
62. Cohen JD, Li L, Wang Y, et al. Detection and localization of surgically resectable cancers with a multi-analyte blood test. Science 2018;359(6378):926–30.
63. Campos-Carrillo A, Weitzel JN, Sahoo P, et al. Circulating tumor DNA as an early cancer detection tool. Pharmacol Ther 2020;207:107458.
64. Colombe P, Béguin J, Benchekroun G, et al. Blood biomarkers for canine cancer, from human to veterinary oncology. Vet Comp Oncol 2022;20(4):767–77.
65. Senhorello ILS, Terra EM, Sueiro FAR, et al. Clinical value of carcinoembryonic antigen in mammary neoplasms of bitches. Vet Comp Oncol 2020;18(3):315–23.
66. Campos LC, Lavalle GE, Estrela-Lima A, et al. CA15.3, CEA and LDH in dogs with malignant mammary tumors. J Vet Intern Med 2012;26(6):1383–8.
67. Fan Y, Ren X, Liu X, et al. Combined detection of CA15-3, CEA, and SF in serum and tissue of canine mammary gland tumor patients. Sci Rep 2021;11(1):6651.
68. Marconato L, Crispino G, Finotello R, et al. Serum lactate dehydrogenase activity in canine malignancies. Vet Comp Oncol 2009;7(4):236–43.
69. Tan HT, Low J, Lim SG, et al. Serum autoantibodies as biomarkers for early cancer detection. FEBS J 2009;276(23):6880–904.
70. Fernández Madrid F. Autoantibodies in breast cancer sera: candidate biomarkers and reporters of tumorigenesis. Cancer Lett 2005;230(2):187–98.
71. Beffagna G, Sammarco A, Bedin C, et al. Circulating cell-free DNA in dogs with mammary tumors: short and long fragments and integrity index. PLoS One 2017;12(1):e0169454.
72. Letendre JA, Goggs R. Measurement of plasma cell-free DNA concentrations in dogs with sepsis, trauma, and neoplasia. J Vet Emerg Crit Care 2017;27(3):307–14.
73. Alborelli I, Generali D, Jermann P, et al. Cell-free DNA analysis in healthy individuals by next-generation sequencing: a proof of concept and technical validation study. Cell Death Dis 2019;10(7):534.
74. Kim J, Bae H, Ahn S, et al. Cell-free DNA as a diagnostic and prognostic biomarker in dogs with tumors. Front Vet Sci 2021;8:735682.
75. Schaefer DM, Forman MA, Kisseberth WC, et al. Quantification of plasma DNA as a prognostic indicator in canine lymphoid neoplasia. Vet Comp Oncol 2007;5(3):145–55.
76. Favaro PF, Stewart SD, McDonald BR, et al. Feasibility of circulating tumor DNA analysis in dogs with naturally occurring malignant and benign splenic lesions. Sci Rep 2022;12(1):6337.

77. Shulman DS, Klega K, Imamovic-Tuco A, et al. Detection of circulating tumour DNA is associated with inferior outcomes in Ewing sarcoma and osteosarcoma: a report from the Children's Oncology Group. Br J Cancer 2018;119(5):615–21.
78. Dolan C, Miller T, Jill J, et al. Characterizing circulating nucleosomes in the plasma of dogs with lymphoma. BMC Vet Res 2021;17(1):276.
79. Wilson-Robles H, Miller T, Jarvis J, et al. Characterizing circulating nucleosomes in the plasma of dogs with hemangiosarcoma. BMC Vet Res 2021;17(1):231.
80. von Euler H, Einarsson R, Olsson U, et al. Serum thymidine kinase activity in dogs with malignant lymphoma: a potent marker for prognosis and monitoring the disease. J Vet Intern Med 2004;18(5):696–702.
81. Wilson-Robles HM, Bygott T, Kelly TK, et al. Evaluation of plasma nucleosome concentrations in dogs with a variety of common cancers and in healthy dogs. BMC Vet Res 2022;18(1):329.
82. Letendre JA, Goggs R. Concentrations of plasma nucleosomes but not cell-free DNA are prognostic in dogs following trauma. Front Vet Sci 2018;5:180.
83. Letendre JA, Goggs R. Determining prognosis in canine sepsis by bedside measurement of cell-free DNA and nucleosomes. J Vet Emerg Crit Care 2018; 28(6):503–11.
84. Burnett DL, Cave NJ, Gedye KR, et al. Investigation of cell-free DNA in canine plasma and its relation to disease. Vet Q 2016;36(3):122–9.
85. Troia R, Giunti M, Calipa S, et al. Cell-free DNA, high-mobility group box-1, and procalcitonin concentrations in dogs with gastric dilatation-volvulus syndrome. Front Vet Sci 2018;5:67.
86. Goggs R. Effect of sample type on plasma concentrations of cell-free DNA and nucleosomes in dogs. Vet Rec Open 2019;6(1):e000357.
87. Martiny P, Goggs R. Biomarker guided diagnosis of septic peritonitis in dogs. Front Vet Sci 2019;6:208.
88. Chibuk J, Flory A, Kruglyak KM, et al. Horizons in veterinary precision oncology: fundamentals of cancer genomics and applications of liquid biopsy for the detection, characterization, and management of cancer in dogs. Front Vet Sci 2021;8:664718.
89. Chen XQ, Stroun M, Magnenat JL, et al. Microsatellite alterations in plasma DNA of small cell lung cancer patients. Nat Med 1996;2(9):1033–5.
90. Nawroz-Danish H, Eisenberger CF, Yoo GH, et al. Microsatellite analysis of serum DNA in patients with head and neck cancer. Int J Cancer 2004;111(1): 96–100.
91. Kruglyak KM, Chibuk J, McLennan L, et al. Blood-based liquid biopsy for comprehensive cancer genomic profiling using next-generation sequencing: an emerging paradigm for non-invasive cancer detection and management in dogs. Front Vet Sci 2021;8:704835.
92. Nikanjam M, Kato S, Kurzrock R. Liquid biopsy: current technology and clinical applications. J Hematol Oncol 2022;15(1):131.
93. Sato Y. Clinical utility of liquid biopsy-based companion diagnostics in the non-small-cell lung cancer treatment. Explor Target Antitumor Ther 2022;3(5): 630–42.
94. Sacher AG, Paweletz C, Dahlberg SE, et al. Prospective validation of rapid plasma genotyping for the detection of EGFR and KRAS mutations in advanced lung cancer. JAMA Oncol 2016;2(8):1014–22.
95. Komiya K, Nakashima C, Nakamura T, et al. Current status and problems of T790M detection, a molecular biomarker of acquired resistance to egfr tyrosine

kinase inhibitors, with liquid biopsy and re-biopsy. Anticancer Res 2018;38(6): 3559–66.

96. 360 G. Physician Insert: Guardant 360 CDx Internet. cited 2023 Aug 23. Available at: https://www.guardantcomplete.com/assets/pdf/Guardant360-CDx-Physician-Insert-US.pdf https://www.guardantcomplete.com/assets/pdf/Guardant360-CDx-Physician-Insert-US.pdf.

97. Foundation Medicine Liquid CDx Technical Information Internet. cited 2023 Aug 23. https://assets.ctfassets.net/w98cd481qyp0/3a8jFw3KUjIU3RWPdcT9Ax/b9a0bd4e46fc41a1b133d730e0dd2326/P190032_S010_F1LCDx_Technical_Label_6JULY_2023_CLEAN1.pdf.

98. Sarhadi VK, Armengol G. Molecular Biomarkers in Cancer. Biomolecules 2022;12(8).

99. Cisneros-Villanueva M, Hidalgo-Pérez L, Rios-Romero M, et al. Cell-free DNA analysis in current cancer clinical trials: a review. Br J Cancer 2022;126(3): 391–400.

100. Heitzer E, Haque IS, Roberts CES, et al. Current and future perspectives of liquid biopsies in genomics-driven oncology. Nat Rev Genet 2019;20(2):71–88.

101. Gerlinger M, Rowan AJ, Horswell S, et al. Intratumor heterogeneity and branched evolution revealed by multiregion sequencing. N Engl J Med 2012; 366(10):883–92.

102. O'Kell AL, Lytle KM, Cohen TA, et al. Clinical experience with next-generation sequencing-based liquid biopsy testing for cancer detection in dogs: a review of 1,500 consecutive clinical cases. J Am Vet Med Assoc 2023;261(6):827–36.

103. Thomas R, Smith KC, Ostrander EA, et al. Chromosome aberrations in canine multicentric lymphomas detected with comparative genomic hybridisation and a panel of single locus probes. Br J Cancer 2003;89(8):1530–7.

104. Richards KL, Suter SE. Man's best friend: what can pet dogs teach us about non-Hodgkin's lymphoma? Immunol Rev 2015;263(1):173–91.

105. Maly V, Maly O, Kolostova K, et al. Circulating tumor cells in diagnosis and treatment of lung cancer. In Vivo 2019;33(4):1027–37.

106. Paoletti C, Muñiz MC, Thomas DG, et al. Development of circulating tumor cell-endocrine therapy index in patients with hormone receptor-positive breast cancer. Clin Cancer Res 2015;21(11):2487–98.

107. Marconato L, Facchinetti A, Zanardello C, et al. Detection and prognostic relevance of circulating and disseminated tumour cell in dogs with metastatic mammary carcinoma: a pilot study. Cancers 2019;11(2).

108. Wright TF, Brisson BA, Belanger CR, et al. Quantification of circulating tumour cells over time in dogs with appendicular osteosarcoma. Vet Comp Oncol 2023;21(3):541–50.

109. Yu W, Hurley J, Roberts D, et al. Exosome-based liquid biopsies in cancer: opportunities and challenges. Ann Oncol 2021;32(4):466–77.

110. Hoshino A, Kim HS, Bojmar L, et al. Extracellular vesicle and particle biomarkers define multiple human cancers. Cell 2020;182(4):1044–61.e18.

111. Eroglu Z, Krinshpun S, Kalashnikova E, et al. Circulating tumor DNA-based molecular residual disease detection for treatment monitoring in advanced melanoma patients. Cancer 2023;129(11):1723–34.

112. Henriksen TV, Tarazona N, Frydendahl A, et al. Circulating tumor DNA in stage III colorectal cancer, beyond minimal residual disease detection, toward assessment of adjuvant therapy efficacy and clinical behavior of recurrences. Clin Cancer Res 2022;28(3):507–17.

113. Christensen E, Birkenkamp-Demtröder K, Sethi H, et al. Early detection of metastatic relapse and monitoring of therapeutic efficacy by ultra-deep sequencing of plasma cell-free DNA in patients with urothelial bladder carcinoma. J Clin Oncol 2019;37(18):1547–57.

114. Kim JJ, Kim HY, Choi Z, et al. In-depth circulating tumor DNA sequencing for prognostication and monitoring in natural killer/T-cell lymphomas. Front Oncol 2023;13:1109715.

115. Kasi PM, Fehringer G, Taniguchi H, et al. Impact of circulating tumor DNA-based detection of molecular residual disease on the conduct and design of clinical trials for solid tumors. JCO Precis Oncol 2022;6:e2100181.

116. Tie J, Cohen JD, Wang Y, et al. Serial circulating tumour DNA analysis during multimodality treatment of locally advanced rectal cancer: a prospective biomarker study. Gut 2019;68(4):663–71.

117. PetDx. Evaluation of OncoK9 for Detection of Residual Disease and Cancer Recurrence in Dogs Internet. 2023 cited 2023 Aug 26. https://assets.petdx.com/m/7b129c182d2ae289/original/Cancer-Monitoring-White-Paper-01092023.pdf.

118. Kilgour E, Rothwell DG, Brady G, et al. Liquid biopsy-based biomarkers of treatment response and resistance. Cancer Cell 2020;37(4):485–95.

119. Iwamoto T, Kajiwara Y, Zhu Y, et al. Biomarkers of neoadjuvant/adjuvant chemotherapy for breast cancer. Chin Clin Oncol 2020;9(3):27.

120. Chen H, Xu C, Fang Z, et al. Cell-free DNA, MicroRNAs, Proteins, and peptides as liquid biopsy biomarkers in prostate cancer and bladder cancer. Methods Mol Biol 2023;2695:165–79.

121. Jung G, Hernández-Illán E, Moreira L, et al. Epigenetics of colorectal cancer: biomarker and therapeutic potential. Nat Rev Gastroenterol Hepatol 2020;17(2):111–30.

122. Saellström S, Sharif H, Jagarlamudi KK, et al. Serum TK1 protein and C-reactive protein correlate to treatment response and predict survival in dogs with hematologic malignancies. Res Vet Sci 2022;145:213–21.

123. Bronkhorst AJ, Ungerer V, Holdenrieder S. Early detection of cancer using circulating tumor DNA: biological, physiological and analytical considerations. Crit Rev Clin Lab Sci 2019;1–17.

124. Holdenrieder S, Dharuman Y, Standop J, et al. Novel serum nucleosomics biomarkers for the detection of colorectal cancer. Anticancer Res 2014;34(5):2357–62.

125. Holdenrieder S. Biomarkers along the continuum of care in lung cancer. Scand J Clin Lab Invest Suppl 2016;245:S40–5.

126. Holdenrieder S, Pagliaro L, Morgenstern D, et al. Clinically meaningful use of blood tumor markers in oncology. BioMed Res Int 2016;2016:9795269.

127. Wittwer C, Boeck S, Heinemann V, et al. Circulating nucleosomes and immunogenic cell death markers HMGB1, sRAGE and DNAse in patients with advanced pancreatic cancer undergoing chemotherapy. Int J Cancer 2013;133(11):2619–30.

128. Wilson-Robles H, Warry E, Miller T, et al, editors. Plasma H3.1 nucleosome concentrations in dogs with various carcinomas. Alicante, Spain: European Society of Veterinary Oncology; 2023.

129. Wilson-Robles H, Warry E, Miller T, et al. Monitoring plasma nucleosome concentrations to measure disease response and progression in dogs with hematopoietic malignancies. PLoS One 2023;18(5):e0281796.

130. Diehl F, Schmidt K, Choti MA, et al. Circulating mutant DNA to assess tumor dynamics. Nat Med 2008;14(9):985–90.
131. Callesen LB, Boysen AK, Andersen CSA, et al. The importance of feasibility assessment in the design of ctDNA guided trials - results from the OPTIPAL II study. Clin Colorectal Cancer 2023.
132. McCleary-Wheeler AL, Fiaux PC, Flesner BK, et al. Next-generation sequencing-based liquid biopsy may be used for detection of residual disease and cancer recurrence monitoring in dogs. Am J Vet Res 2023;1–8.
133. Katogiritis A, Khanna C. Towards the delivery of precision veterinary cancer medicine. Vet Clin North Am Small Anim Pract 2019;49(5):809–18.

Update in Veterinary Radiation Oncology

Focus on Stereotactic Radiation Therapy

Michael W. Nolan, DVM, PhD*, Tracy L. Gieger, DVM

KEYWORDS

- Radiotherapy • Stereotactic radiosurgery • Brain tumors • Nasal tumors
- Osteosarcoma • Soft tissue sarcomas • Radiobiology

KEY POINTS

- Stereotactic radiation therapy (SRT) requires accurate and precise delivery of large radiation doses to a well-defined target in a few treatment sessions.
- Common aliases include stereotactic radiosurgery, stereotactic body radiotherapy, stereotactic ablative body radiotherapy, radiosurgery, CyberKnife, and Gamma Knife.
- SRT is increasingly accessible and can be delivered with palliative or definitive intent.
- Common indications include nasal, brain, and appendicular tumors. Emerging uses include oral, lung, prostate, and adrenal tumors.
- Even when technically feasible, SRT is not always the optimal radiation treatment modality.

INTRODUCTION

Few dogs and cats with cancer are treated with radiotherapy (RT) despite increasing availability.[1] Pet owners cite finances, the distance required to travel to veterinary RT centers, protracted treatment schedules, and potential displeasing side effects as deterrents. Stereotactic RT (SRT) overcomes several of these barriers. With SRT, large doses of radiation are carefully sculpted to match the shape of the target (tumor) and then delivered with exacting precision. This allows intensive courses of cancer treatment to be compressed into five or fewer treatment sessions, often with minimal acute toxicity. The purpose of this article is to review the key features of SRTs unique radiobiology, describe the evidence base for common and emerging applications of SRT applications, and discuss controversies in the use of SRT.

Department of Clinical Sciences, College of Veterinary Medicine, North Carolina State University, 1060 William Moore Drive, Raleigh, NC 27607, USA
* Corresponding author.
E-mail address: mwnolan@ncsu.edu

Vet Clin Small Anim 54 (2024) 559–575
https://doi.org/10.1016/j.cvsm.2023.12.009
0195-5616/24/© 2023 Elsevier Inc. All rights reserved.

PHYSICS AND BIOLOGY OF STEREOTACTIC RADIOTHERAPY

SRT involves the delivery of large fractional doses of radiation to a well-defined target with extreme accuracy (stereotaxis) and with a steep radiation dose gradient that escalates the dose in the target while minimizing the dose in adjacent healthy tissues.

A variety of technologies have been developed for SRT planning and delivery. Beginning in 1951, Lars Leksell developed the Gamma Knife system, which combines a stereotactic headframe with 179 sealed cobalt-60 sources that can be collimated to produce favorable radiation dose distributions.[2,3] The Gamma Knife remains in use today. CyberKnife represents another approach, wherein a 6-MV linear accelerator (linac) is mounted on a robotic arm that can literally dance around the patient. Hundreds of small radiation beamlets are delivered from multiple angles and converge on the tumor, whose location is verified with submillimeter accuracy by matching bony landmarks and/or intratumoral gold fiducial markers using orthogonal radiography. Conventional C-arm linacs can also be modified to allow SRT. The best-accepted methodology involves use of either intensity-modulated RT (IMRT), or volumetric-modulated arc therapy plans to achieve adequate conformity and dose gradients and cone beam CT (CBCT)-based image guidance to achieve stereotaxis. Regardless of the mechanisms used for treatment planning and delivery, equipment that is designed for SRT will generally produce similar dosimetric and clinical outcomes.

In addition to the various mechanical SRT systems, several acronyms are also used to describe this therapeutic modality. Stereotactic radiosurgery (SRS) refers to a single fraction protocol, often limited to a central nervous system target. Stereotactic body RT (SBRT) refers to the treatment of a non-central nervous system (CNS) target.[2] The term "stereotactic ablative body radiotherapy" reflects the notion that targeted, high-dose radiation can be used to "ablate" a tissue (ie, render it nonfunctional). This concept is founded in the radiobiologic basis of SRT and how it is thought to differ from conventional, finely fractionated RT (FRT).[3]

In classic radiobiology, DNA is considered the target of ionizing radiation. Unrepaired DNA double-strand breaks halt tumor growth by preventing cell cycle progression and/or inducing cell death. In clinical practice, a margin of normal tissue has conventionally been included in the treatment field to account for microscopic tumor extension, and an additional margin is used to account for inter- and intra-fraction motion, comprising the planning target volume (PTV). A homogeneous dose of radiation is then prescribed to the PTV. Even with highly conformal treatment plans, this approach results in the delivery of equal doses of radiation to both tumor and normal tissues within the PTV. In FRT, the repair of sublethal DNA damage and repopulation of cells between radiation fractions protect normal tissues. Between doses of FRT, reoxygenation of previously hypoxic tumor and redistribution of surviving tumor cells to more sensitive phases of the cell cycle enhance tumor control. The impact of these 4 R's (repair, repopulation, reoxygenation, redistribution) can be seen in experiments performed to determine radiation dose–response relationships in vitro. Resultant cell survival curves can be mathematically modeled. The linear–quadratic (LQ) model predicts that for any given dose of radiation, delivery via large fractional doses will be associated with a higher risk of severe late radiation toxicity than if the dose had been given in multiple smaller dose fractions. This is particularly true in certain so-called late-responding normal tissues, such as the spinal cord, heart, bones, and peripheral nerves, all characterized by a low alpha-to-beta ratio. Rather than biological sparing, SRT excludes as much normal tissue from the planning target volume (PTV) as possible and physically shields tissues that are immediately adjacent. This approach enables delivery of large dose fractions (>6 Gy, vs 2.5–3 Gy fractions that are typically used in FRT). Interestingly, clinical and experimental outcomes of SRT often exceed that which would be predicted by LQ modeling. Regardless of whether one trusts the LQ model in the setting of severely hypofractionated RT (>6–8 Gy fractions), it is increasingly clear that ionizing radiation has differential effects at high versus low fractional doses.

SRT biology is perhaps most unique in the tumor microenvironment. Fuks and Kolesnickdemonstrated that high-dose irradiation induces endothelial cell acid sphingomyelinase translocation, which hydrolyzes sphingomyelin to generate ceramide, thus initiating apoptosis and microvascular collapse.[4] Their results have not been replicated, and conflicting data call into question the importance of this endothelial response.[5] Regardless of mechanism, numerous other reports describe severe vascular destruction and dysfunction at doses of $\geq$ 10 Gy in experimental rodent tumors.[6,7] This vascular dysfunction causes tumor hypoxia that can impair homologous recombination repair of radiation-induced DNA double-strand breaks and produce secondary cell killing.[8] In addition to vascular effects, it is also well established that radiation induces immunogenic cell death and primes T cells to tumor antigens.[9,10] The magnitude and character of these effects are influenced by radiation dose, and interestingly, the "optimal" immunogenic dose of radiation is not necessarily the highest radiation dose.[11] Recent preclinical data indicate that systemic effects of localized radiation are mediated by CD8+ T cells and interferon receptors, but that one or three daily doses of 8 Gy improve outcomes as compared with single doses of 20 to 30 Gy or less than 8 Gy.[12]

Independent of tumor microenvironment effects, high radiation dose intensity is another key difference between SRT and FRT. Large (6–9 Gy) dose fractions have long been used in palliative care for veterinary patients, but those fractions have most often been delivered at 7-day intervals. Even though the size of SRT dose fractions is similar, SRT uses much shorter (24–48 hour) intrafraction intervals. This difference is impactful because tumors are continually growing. Hence, reduction in total treatment time reduces the number of tumor cells that are "seen" by a given dose of radiation, thus improving the expected efficacy of treatment on a per-Gray basis.

CLINICAL APPROACH TO STEREOTACTIC RADIOTHERAPY

The key components of SRT include: (1) clinical evaluation to ensure suitability, (2) optimizing patient immobilization and respiratory motion to enable reproducible positioning, (3) delineating tumor versus non-tumor compartments via imaging, (4) treatment planning that generates steep dose gradients between organs at risk (OAR) and target tissues, and (5) verification of precise patient position via on-board imaging, before (6) accurate dose delivery.[4] In veterinary medicine, the use of SRT is largely anecdotal, with recent publications focusing on a few specific tumor types.

CLINICAL DATA: BRAIN TUMORS

Canine and feline brain tumors are frequently treated with SRT; recent publications have documented outcomes for individual tumor types (**Table 1**). Survival times are generally similar when comparing SRT and FRT, but it remains unclear whether SRT causes more toxicity. Two publications report that approximately one-third of dogs receiving SRT for intracranial meningioma experience neurologic decline in the first 6 months after treatment.[13,14] Although most dogs in those studies improved (typically with steroid administration), these events were sometimes fatal. In most cases, early-delayed radiation toxicity was suspected, as opposed to tumor progression, but this could not be confirmed due to the lack of reimaging and/or necropsy (**Fig. 1**). It is

Table 1
Summary of recent publications regarding stereotactic radiotherapy for intracranial tumors in dogs

Reference	Tumor Type	# Dogs	Radiation Prescription(s)	Overall Survival Time	Toxicity	Comments
Hansen et al,[63] 2023	Intraventricular tumors	11	8 Gy × 3 = 24 Gy 15 Gy × 1 = 15 Gy	Median 151 d (95% CI 33–1593)	None reported; 2 dogs were euthanized within 6 wk of SRT	6/11 had biopsy confirmation of choroid plexus papilloma or carcinoma or ependymoma
Carter et al,[64] 2021	Intracranial tumors	59	7–8.5 Gy × 3 = 21–25.5 Gy	Median 738 d	None reported	Progression-free survival varied by location: cerebrum 357 d, cerebellum 97 d, brainstem 266 d; overall median ST of dogs with presumed meningiomas was not reached at > 2079 d
Moirano et al,[65] 2020	Glioma	21	8–9.5 Gy × 3 = 24–27 Gy	Median 636 d	3/21 had presumed acute toxicity that responded to steroids	7/21 had additional courses of SRT, and median ST of those dogs was 866 d
Swift et al,[66] 2017	Trigeminal nerve sheath tumor	27 dogs (15 treated with SRT)	8 Gy × 3 = 24 Gy 10 Gy × 3 = 30 Gy	Median 441 d (95% CI 260–518) for dogs treated with SRT	Some dogs developed facial pain after treatment	Owing to overlap in the 95% CI between treated and untreated dogs, unknown benefit of SRT as compared with no treatment; clinical signs such as facial pain and ocular deficits did not resolve after treatment in most dogs

Study	Tumor	N	Dose	Survival	Toxicity	Notes
Dolera et al,[67] 2018	Trigeminal nerve sheath tumor	7	7.4 Gy × 5 = 37 Gy	Median 952 d (95% CI, 543–1361 d)	None reported	MRI after radiotherapy in all dogs; 1 CR, 4 PR, 2 SD; 4/7 dogs had extracranial extension of the tumor; clinical signs did not resolve in most dogs.
Hansen et al,[68] 2016	Trigeminal nerve sheath tumor	8	8 Gy × 3 = 24 Gy	Median 324 days (95% CI: 99–975)	None reported. 6/8 dogs were euthanized due to seizures and progressive neurologic signs, and the remaining two dogs experienced accident-related death	Median disease-specific survival time: 745 d
Dolera et al,[69] 2018	Glioma	42	4.2 Gy × 10 = 42 Gy 5.3 Gy × 7 = 37 Gy 6.6 Gy × 5 = 33 Gy 7 Gy × 5 = 35 Gy	RT alone: 50% alive at 1 y, 41% at 2 y RT + TMZ: 65% alive at 1 y, 40% at 2 y	Minimal	Radiation dose was scaled based on tumor grade and volume 22 dogs RT alone; 20 RT + temozolomide (TMZ); no difference in outcomes; RT dose based on size of tumor relative to normal brain
Griffin et al,[14] 2016	Meningioma	30	8 Gy × 3 = 24 Gy	Median 561 d (95% CI 423–875d), 60.8% at 1 y survival, 33.2% 2 y	37% worsened neurologically 3–16 wk after SRT; 13% died of neurologic progression within 6 mo	Volume of normal brain treated predicted death

(continued on next page)

Table 1
(continued)

Reference	Tumor Type	# Dogs	Radiation Prescription(s)	Overall Survival Time	Toxicity	Comments
Kelsey et al,[13] 2018	Meningioma	32	16 Gy x 1 = 16 Gy	Median 519 d (95% CI 330–708d), 64% 1 y survival, 24% 2 y	31% worsened neurologically within 6 months after SRT; 10% died of neuro progression	Infratentorial tumors and higher gradient index predicted shorter survival time
Dolera et al,[70] 2018	Meningioma	39 (33 with encephalic meningioma, 6 spinal meningioma)	6.6 Gy × 5 = 33 Gy	2-y overall survival: 74.3%	One dog had mild neurotoxicity	2-year disease-specific survival: 97.4%. 49% of dogs had a partial or complete response at 2 years, when considering both objective follow-up imaging data and clinical status in response evaluation.

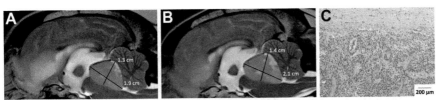

Fig. 1. In the absence of cross-sectional imaging to prove tumor progression, neurologic decline within the first few months after SRT/SRS is typically attributed to early-delayed neuro-radiotoxicity in retrospective studies. Objective data are needed to better characterize outcomes. (*A*) A midbrain tumor that was treated with SRS. The dog's neurologic signs worsened a month after SRS and failed to improve with symptomatic treatment for early-delayed neurotoxicity. (*B*) Recheck MRI 2 months after SRS revealed tumor enlargement. Progression and pseudoprogression were differential diagnoses. (*C*) Necropsy revealed ependymoma without intratumoral edema, inflammation or degeneration, and without radiation-induced changes in adjacent neuroparenchyma. (*Courtesy of* Dr Marc Kent, DVM, University of Georgia, Athens, GA.)

critical that practitioners treating brain tumors with SRT continue working to identify predictors of toxicity and oncologic response. Future studies should ideally include regularly scheduled and prospectively collected neurologic outcomes assessments/surveys and follow-up imaging, and increased use of necropsy that clinical findings can be correlated with imaging and histopathology data.

Beyond the published data, it is notable that non-resectable and recurrent intracranial feline meningiomas can be treated with SRT. In addition to primary brain tumors, feline pituitary masses can also be irradiated. These tumors often cause acromegaly with insulin-resistant diabetes mellitus (DM), and two studies (one describing 53 cats treated with 17–28 Gy given over 3–4 fractions, and the other including 14 cats treated with a single fraction of 17 Gy) have yielded similar results.[15,16] Impressively, of these cats, 95% and 71% (respectively) had decreased insulin requirements. The median time to lowest insulin dose was 9.5 to 13 months, and 21% to 32% achieved complete diabetic remission. Adverse events were typically mild; in one of these reports, hypothyroidism developed after SRT in 14% of the cats.[15] The overall median survival times for the two groups of cats were 1072 and 741 days, respectively. Dogs also develop functional and nonfunctional pituitary tumors, which are discussed in the following.

CLINICAL DATA: HEAD AND NECK CANCER

External beam megavoltage RT is the cornerstone of management for canine non-lymphomatous sinonasal tumors. A recent systematic review found that conventional palliative-intent RT protocols were associated with median overall survival times ranging from 4.8 to 16.8 months (median 8.5 months), whereas survival ranged from 10.4 to 19.1 months (median 14.0 months) after treatment with definitive-intent FRT.[17]

SRT is increasingly used. A major appeal is that treatment causes few/mild acute side effects, and treatment courses are succinct. Early reports were encouraging,[18–21] and in the largest published data set (a group of 129 dogs treated with 30 Gy total in 3 fractions), the median overall survival time was 18 months. A significant advantage may arise when considering treatment of dogs with advanced local disease; with SRT, survival often exceeds a year even when tumors invade the cranial vault; this is in contrast to conventional RT, where median survival times are 6 to 7 months with cribriform lysis.[22–24]

As long-term survivorship improves, careful attention must be paid to maximizing quality of life. Dogs who gain excellent tumor control from SRT are at risk for developing one or more significant complications of either the disease or its treatment. For example, many dogs will experience chronic rhinosinusitis that develops secondary to tumor and/or radiation-induced damage to the mucociliary apparatus (**Fig. 2**). Other dogs may develop osteoradionecrosis and/or dermal atrophy with subsequent forma-tion of either oronasal or nasocutaneous fistulae. Careful documentation will help deter-mine the actual risk of such complications, and formal scientific investigation is needed to develop strategies that effectively prevent or treat these conditions.

Beyond the growing acceptance of SRT as the most ideal treatment option currently available for managing most cases of canine intranasal malignancies, there are also published data to support the use of SRT as a re-treatment option for recurrent and

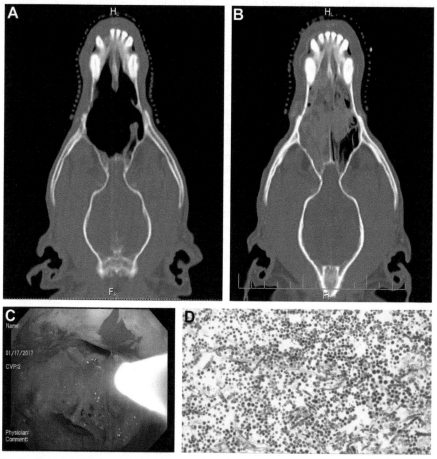

Fig. 2. Chronic rhinitis and sinusitis are relatively common in dogs with nasal tumors that have excellent tumor control after SRT. Sterile inflammation is possible, but secondary infec-tion (with or without osteomyelitis) must also be considered. (*A*) A nasal carcinoma that was treated with SRT. Clinical signs improved, but nasal discharge recurred 22 months later. (*B*) Recheck CT revealed complete resolution of the tumor with progressive osteolysis and com-plete loss of the nasal septum. (*C*) Rhinoscopy revealed plaques. (*D*) Histopathology revealed pigmented fungal spores and hyphae. Infection resolved with clotrimazole infusions.

progressive canine nasal tumors,[25] as well as in a wide range of other head and neck malignancies including intranasal lymphomas[26] and carcinomas[27] of the cat, as well as feline facial squamous cell carcinomas,[28] canine salivary gland carcinomas,[29] and canine thyroid tumors.[30]

CLINICAL DATA: THORACIC AND ABDOMINAL CAVITY MALIGNANCIES

Intrathoracic tumors present a unique challenge for RT planning and delivery due to constant cardiac and thoracic cavity movement and intimate association of tumors with the great vessels, trachea, esophagus, and heart (which are generally very tolerant of FRT, but become dose-limiting in SRT). The process of RT planning begins with a CT scan, for which considerations to delineate OAR (such as the esophagus, which may be delineated with assistance of a radiopaque esophageal feeding tube) as well as management of respiratory motion (using techniques such as high-frequency jet ventilation or respiratory neuroparalytics and breath holding) should be made in advance of the scan.[31]

There is a paucity of literature documenting outcomes with irradiation of intrathoracic tumors in veterinary patients, and a gold standard for treatment of nonsurgically resectable tumors does not exist. In an early study, six dogs with presumed or confirmed chemodectomas were treated with SBRT (30 Gy in 3 fractions delivered in 3–5 days).[32] Treatments were planned with IMRT, and CBCT was used to verify patient positioning before irradiation. Respiratory motion was managed with neuroparalytics (or jet ventilation [approximately 180 breaths/minute]). The tumor volume decreased by 30% to 70% in all four dogs that were re-imaged after treatment. Possible treatment-associated toxicities included periprocedural esophageal reflux, cough, tachyarrhythmias, and congestive heart failure. Two dogs died suddenly at 150 and 294 days after SBRT, and the other four lived greater than 408 days after treatment. Arrhythmias, heart failure, and sudden death may have been attributable to the tumor or radiation injury to the heart. However, in a more recent publication, a similar SBRT protocol was used to treat 26 dogs, and there were no irradiation-induced adverse cardiac events observed.[33] Beyond this, the only other intrathoracic disease for which there are published outcomes data is canine thymoma; in a recent publication describing outcomes for 15 dogs, survival was similar, but toxicity was improved when SRT was used instead of conventional non-modulated RT.[34] Other intrathoracic diseases that have been treated with SBRT at our institution include intrathoracic sarcomas, primary lung tumors, oligometastatic lung tumors, and cardiac hemangiosarcomas. Of note, patients with pleural or pericardial effusion may not be candidates for SBRT because dynamic changes in fluid volumes over the course of treatment can affect dosimetry of radiation treatment plans and respiratory motion management.

Abdomino-pelvic malignancies are also increasingly managed with SBRT. As with the thorax, respiratory motion and proximity to critical normal tissues must be carefully considered for cranial abdominal tumors. In a recent publication describing SBRT for canine adrenocortical tumors, three of nine dogs had cortisol-secreting tumors, and six of nine tumors were discovered incidentally.[35] Radiation prescriptions ranged from 30 to 45 Gy in 3 to 5 daily fractions; dose escalations were made based on proximity of the target to OAR. To limit thoracic excursions, the dogs were positioned in lateral recumbency, and the abdomen was taped during treatment. For planning, an internal margin (IM) was calculated by determining displacement of the gross tumor volume (GTV) between maximum inspiration and expiration. A setup margin was added to the IM + GTV to create a PTV. No significant side effects were noted. Whole body CT scans were performed 2, 4, and 6 months after SBRT. All dogs had progressive tumor size reduction, with a mean decrease in diameter and volume of 32% and 30%, respectively. The overall median survival time following treatment was 1030 days. Similar results have been observed in dogs undergoing SBRT for pheochromocytoma.[36] In that report, dogs were treated with 11 Gy × 3 consecutive daily fractions when tumors were small and distant from the alimentary tract or 7 Gy × 5 every-other-day fractions when large and abutting gastrointestinal organs. All dogs were pretreated with phenoxybenzamine. Adverse events were rare, and five of eight dogs were alive at the time of publication, with a median follow-up time of 25.8 months. Based on these results, SBRT seems to be a reasonable alternative to surgical management of adrenal tumors, even when there is extensive vascular invasion or clinically worrisome endocrine activity. Anecdotally, we have achieved clinical benefit by treatment of retroperitoneal sarcomas, solitary hepatocellular carcinoma, renal cell carcinoma, and prostate-confined neoplasms with SBRT, and there is also a recent case report suggesting that prolonged survival can be achievable with minimal treatment-induced morbidity in dogs with anal sac adenocarcinomas, even when there is extensive lymph node metastasis.[37]

Duration of the interfraction interval is an important consideration for abdominopelvic irradiation. Men with prostate cancer are frequently treated with 5-fraction SBRT protocols, to a total of 35 to 36.25 Gy. Their risk of late colorectal complication is decreased by separation of radiation dose fractions by at least 36 hours,[38] that is done without any apparent impact on tumor control. Similar risk reduction has been reported for dogs and is achieved by decreasing the likelihood of a consequential late effect (ie, the unusual situation wherein a late effect arises secondary to a severe acute effect).[39,40] Recall, however, that total treatment time is not a recognized risk factor for classic late toxicities. Thus, although prolongation of the interfraction interval may prove beneficial for patients when the tumor abuts acutely responding tissue, and when the requisite dose for tumor control exceeds the tolerance of that normal tissue, this strategy is unlikely to provide benefit for patients undergoing SRT at sites such as the brain.

CLINICAL DATA: OSTEOSARCOMA

Although the "gold standard" for treatment of osteosarcoma (OSA) remains complete surgical excision followed by chemotherapy, RT can be an appealing alternative in certain cases. The use of high fractional doses in SBRT may theoretically provide improved tumor control versus FRT because OSA is thought to be a tumor with a low alpha-to-beta ratio and may in fact provide a locally curative limb-salvage option.[41,42] Most suitable for SBRTs are those dogs who are poor candidates for limb amputation or whose owners decline amputation.

SRT anecdotally provides potent and lasting analgesia in a majority of dogs with appendicular OSA. When SRT is combined with chemotherapy, survival is comparable to that achieved with amputation plus carboplatin.[43–45] Interestingly, higher radiation doses seem to be associated with longer overall survival.[45] Aside from distant metastasis, the biggest concern is early treatment failure due to pathologic limb fracture. Early reports raised particular concern about this. In a 2016 paper from the University of Florida, 29 of 46 dogs (63%) developed fractures after SRT,[44] and the institution published data warning against prophylactic surgical stabilization of limbs due to high rates of complications.[46] However, in a larger and more recent study, fracture was only observed in 51 of 123 dogs (41%). Regardless, careful case selection is paramount, and in that regard, clinicians should consider that risk of pathologic fracture increases with the severity of cortical bone lysis, and when there is subchondral bone lysis.[44,47]

It is also a reasonable option for non-resectable axial bone tumors. A recent case series describes nine dogs with primary or metastatic vertebral OSA that were treated with SRT (13.5–36 Gy in 1–5 fractions).[48] Five of six dogs with spinal pain experienced analgesia, with a median clinical response duration of 77 days. The overall survival time for these nine dogs was 139 days. The investigators acknowledged the difficulty of trying to dosimetrically spare the spinal cord adjacent to the tumor (to reduce risk of radiation-induced myelopathy as a potential late effect) while simultaneously delivering a dose of RT that would be sufficient to afford durable tumor control. Although standard dose tolerance recommendations are often used in SBRT prescriptions, recent animal model data suggest that those recommendations may be too conservative and that cautious dose escalation for spinal tumors should be tolerable.[49,50]

CONTROVERSIES IN STEREOTACTIC RADIOTHERAPY

There are significant differences of opinion regarding optimal application of SRT. Here, the authors summarize some of the most interesting controversies.

What Is the Minimum Requirement for Safe and Effective Stereotactic Radiotherapy Delivery?

A growing number of veterinary RT centers have acquired equipment that is designed for SRT planning and delivery. Other centers are meeting the demand by adapting and upgrading older technologies.[51] It is important for clinicians to be aware that it is not simply a matter of combining IMRT with image guidance that enables SRT. SRT treatments require different quality assurance tests and linac tolerances; for example, per the American Association of Physicists in Medicine Task Group report 142, stricter tolerance limits exist for imaging (eg, CBCT), couch position indicators and lasers, and coincidence of the mechanical and radiation isocenters for SRS/SBRT versus non-SRS/SBRT.[52] In addition, target dose conformity and steepness of dose gradients that are acceptable for full-course IMRT may be insufficient for SRT. There is also new anatomy that needs to be learned. For example, the optic chiasm is not commonly contoured for full-course RT but is routinely drawn for SRT of certain calvarial targets. Guidelines for normal tissue contouring are increasingly available to aid practitioners as they learn SRT planning.[53] Finally, although planar imaging may be sufficient for localization of certain osseous targets, the limitations of such imaging must be carefully considered. For example, the prostate translates in the cranial-to-caudal direction depending on bladder filling. Thus, the use of the pelvic bones as a surrogate for prostate location would be insufficient, unless a large expansion of the target volume were used to account for substantial potential setup error. This could be overcome by using intratumorally implanted fiducial markers.

Can Stereotactic Radiotherapy Be Used to Effectively Manage Residual Microscopic Disease Burdens After Surgery?

Conventional FRT is often used after surgery for treatment of brain tumors, cutaneous mast cell tumors and soft tissue sarcomas, and oral tumors. Depending on the tumor and patient characteristics, RT fields are usually drawn to encompass the surgical bed plus 1 to 4 cm of surrounding normal tissue. FRT dosing is based on normal tissue tolerance. Some veterinary radiation oncologists now offer SRT in such cases, using ablative doses for large fields that contain mostly normal tissue, and just a few residual tumor cells.[1] In a study of 36 dogs with grade II and III marginally or incompletely excised soft tissue sarcomas, a liquid fiducial marker was used to delineate the surgical field and a single fraction of 20 Gy was delivered.[54] The local recurrence rate was

24%, with a median time to recurrence of 272 days. Six of those dogs (16.7%) had grade 3 acute skin toxicity, with one requiring wound debridement and a skin flap to address necrosis. Based on clinical outcomes that were similar to those expected with conventional FRT, the authors proposed the continued use of this treatment protocol.[54] Other practitioners remain skeptical, with concern that with such approaches, uncomplicated tumor control will be compromised by either excessive toxicity or excessive tumor recurrence resulting from application of total radiation doses that are too low or radiation fields that are too small. It is also important to ask: if SRT works via unique radiobiological effects in the tumor microenvironment, is it possible to capitalize on those effects in the absence of a bulky tumor?

Are There Bulky Tumors that Make Poor Stereotactic Radiotherapy Candidates?

The highly infiltrative and large nature of most canine nasal tumors suggests that they would not be ideal SRT candidates; however, published data regarding linac-based SRT are encouraging.[21] Conversely, pituitary macroadenomas are often thought of as an ideal target for SRT. Iindeed, the use of SRT for management of feline acromegaly has been rewarding.[15,16] However, initial experiences regarding SRT for management of canine pituitary macroadenomas are more worrisome. In two studies (N = 13 dogs treated with 16 Gy in a single fraction[55] and N = 41 dogs treated with 8 Gy × 3 or 15 Gy × 1[56]), median survival times were 357 and 311, which does not compare favorably with previously published estimates of survival in nonirradiated dogs (median overall survival time 359 days in a group of 27 dogs).[57] This is interesting because (1) these tumors are extra-axial and usually well demarcated on cross-sectional imaging, thus there is no real concern for invasion into surrounding neuroparenchyma; (2) they are encased within a bony target and thus simple to localize for treatment; and (3) they are usually round/spherical, which simplifies the process of generating a treatment plan that is highly conformal and has steep dose gradients. Nevertheless, based on currently available data, caution is recommended when considering 1- and 3-fraction SRT for canine pituitary tumors. A recent abstract suggests that 5-fraction SRT may be more beneficial; there were no differences in outcome for dogs treated with SRT (30 or 35 Gy total in 5 daily fractions) versus FRT (50–54 Gy in 19 or 20 daily fractions), and the median survival time for both groups exceeded 600 days.[58]

Canine soft tissue sarcomas form bulky tumors that are usually successfully managed with surgery (with or without adjunctive RT). However, surgical alternatives can be desirable. In this scenario, conventional hypofractionated palliative-intent RT is commonly used.[59,60] However, SRT may be more effective (**Fig. 3**). In one study of dogs treated with 2 or 3 fractions totaling 27 to 48 Gy, a 46% overall response rate was noted, and the median tumor progression-free interval was 521 days with an overall median survival time of 713 days.[61] Dogs with extremity tumors and those with lower tumor grades had better outcomes, indicating a need for continued study on which patients comprise the most "ideal" treatment group. A similar study using total doses of 20 to 30 Gy delivered in 1 to 5 fractions yielded an overall survival time of 228 days with a disease progression-free survival of 173 days.[62] In that study, dogs with larger tumors were at higher risk of disease progression. Higher skin doses were associated with increased side effects, and 11% of dogs experienced grade three acute dermatoradiotoxicity.

FUTURE DIRECTIONS

Veterinary radiation oncology has undergone incredible growth regarding adoption of new SRT technologies and protocols. This has been mirrored by increases in the

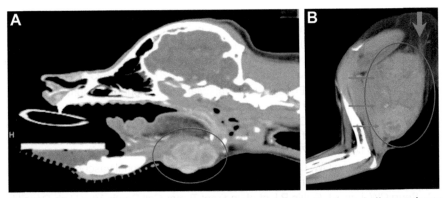

Fig. 3. Treatment of soft tissue sarcomas with RT alone can present unique challenges due to their size and location. Ideally, when SRT is a consideration, a tumor should be well demarcated and contrast-enhancing on CT scan to delineate it from surrounding normal tissues. (A) This soft tissue sarcoma on the mandible of a dog (*circled*) is contrast-enhancing and well demarcated from the surrounding tissues. (B) This soft tissue sarcoma on the forelimb of a dog (*circled*) is minimally contrast-enhancing, and its wispy margins (*thick arrow*) and poor demarcation from the adjacent muscle (*thin arrows*) make it challenging to define when considering highly focused SRT.

amount of published data describing initial clinical experiences with SRT for various diseases. Yet, questions regarding appropriate application of this unique treatment modality still abound. Future studies would ideally focus on further defining recommended OAR dose constraints, as well as long-term outcomes for treated patients. As long-term survivorship improves, we will need significant effort devoted to timely identification of strategies that maximize quality of life in patients who are already enjoying extended quantity of life.

CLINICS CARE POINTS

- SRT is an attractive option that can replace conventional full-course radiotherapy with a succinct treatment course that is completed in 5 or fewer treatment session.
- With SRT, acute side effects are generally quite mild, if at all present.
- For some tumor types, SRT may be more effective than conventional radiotherapy; examples include canine intranasal tumors and extremity osteosarcoma.
- For other tumors and clinical scenarios, an appropriate role for SRT has yet to be defined; examples include incompletely excised tumors.

DISCLOSURE

The authors have no relevant commercial or financial conflicts of interest or funding sources which are relevant to this article.

REFERENCES

1. Dunfield EM, Turek MM, Buhr KA, et al. A survey of stereotactic radiation therapy in veterinary medicine. Vet Radiol Ultrasound 2018;59(6):786–95.

2. Yang M, Timmerman R. Stereotactic ablative radiotherapy uncertainties: delineation, setup and motion. Semin Radiat Oncol 2018;28(3):207–17.

3. Brown JM, Carlson DJ, Brenner DJ. Dose escalation, not "new biology," can account for the efficacy of stereotactic body radiation therapy with non-small cell lung cancer reply. Int J Radiat Oncol Biol Phys 2014;89(3):693–4.

4. Fuks Z, Kolesnick R. Engaging the vascular component of the tumor response. Cancer Cell 2005;8(2):89–91.

5. Moding EJ, Castle KD, Perez BA, et al. Tumor cells, but not endothelial cells, mediate eradication of primary sarcomas by stereotactic body radiation therapy. Sci Transl Med 2015;7(278):278ra34.

6. Wong HH, Song CW, Levitt SH. Early changes in functional vasculature of Walker carcinoma 256 following irradiation. Radiology 1973;108(2):429–34.

7. Song CW, Lee YJ, Griffin RJ, et al. Indirect Tumor Cell Death After High-Dose Hypofractionated Irradiation: Implications for Stereotactic Body Radiation Therapy and Stereotactic Radiation Surgery. Int J Radiat Oncol Biol Phys 2015;93(1):166–72.

8. Kumareswaran R, Ludkovski O, Meng A, et al. Chronic hypoxia compromises repair of DNA double-strand breaks to drive genetic instability. J Cell Sci 2012;125(1):189–99.

9. Stone HB, Peters LJ, Milas L. Effect of host immune capability on radiocurability and subsequent transplantability of a murine fibrosarcoma. J Natl Cancer Inst 1979;63(5):1229–35.

10. Lugade AA, Moran JP, Gerber SA, et al. Local radiation therapy of B16 melanoma tumors increases the generation of tumor antigen-specific effector cells that traffic to the tumor. J Immunol 2005;174(12):7516–23.

11. Dewan MZ, Galloway AE, Kawashima N, et al. Fractionated but not single-dose radiotherapy induces an immune-mediated abscopal effect when combined with anti-CTLA-4 antibody. Clin Cancer Res 2009;15(17):5379–88.

12. Vanpouille-Box C, Alard A, Aryankalayil MJ, et al. DNA exonuclease Trex1 regulates radiotherapy-induced tumour immunogenicity. Nat Commun 2017;8:15618.

13. Kelsey KL, Gieger TL, Nolan MW. Single fraction stereotactic radiation therapy (stereotactic radiosurgery) is a feasible method for treating intracranial meningiomas in dogs. Vet Radiol Ultrasound 2018;59(5):632–8.

14. Griffin LR, Nolan MW, Selmic LE, et al. Stereotactic radiation therapy for treatment of canine intracranial meningiomas. Vet Comp Oncol 2016;14(4):E158–70.

15. Wormhoudt TL, Boss MK, Lunn K, et al. Stereotactic radiation therapy for the treatment of functional pituitary adenomas associated with feline acromegaly. J Vet Intern Med 2018;32(4):1383–91.

16. Watson-Skaggs ML, Gieger TL, Yoshikawa H, et al. Endocrine response and outcome in 14 cats with insulin resistance and acromegaly treated with stereotactic radiosurgery (17 Gy). Am J Vet Res 2021;83(1):64–71.

17. Nolan MW, Dobson JM. The future of radiotherapy in small animals - should the fractions be coarse or fine? J Small Anim Pract 2018;59(9):521–30.

18. Fox-Alvarez S, Shiomitsu K, Lejeune AT, et al. Outcome of intensity-modulated radiation therapy-based stereotactic radiation therapy for treatment of canine nasal carcinomas. Vet Radiol Ultrasound 2020;61(3):370–8.

19. Mayer MN, DeWalt JO, Sidhu N, et al. Outcomes and adverse effects associated with stereotactic body radiation therapy in dogs with nasal tumors: 28 cases (2011–2016). J Am Vet Med Assoc 2019;254(5):602–12.

20. Glasser SA, Charney S, Dervisis NG, et al. Use of an image-guided robotic radio-surgery system for the treatment of canine nonlymphomatous nasal tumors. J Am Anim Hosp Assoc 2014;50(2):96–104.
21. Gieger TL, Nolan MW. Linac-based stereotactic radiation therapy for canine non-lymphomatous nasal tumours: 29 cases (2013-2016). Vet Comp Oncol 2018; 16(1):E68–75.
22. Lawrence JA, Forrest LJ, Turek MM, et al. Proof of principle of ocular sparing in dogs with sinonasal tumors treated with intensity-modulated radiation therapy. Vet Radiol Ultrasound 2010;51(5):561–70.
23. Adams WM, Miller PE, Vail DM, et al. An accelerated technique for irradiation of malignant canine nasal and paranasal sinus tumors. Vet Radiol Ultrasound 1998; 39(5):475–81.
24. Adams WM, Kleiter MM, Thrall DE, et al. Prognostic significance of tumor histol-ogy and computed tomographic staging for radiation treatment response of canine nasal tumors. Vet Radiol Ultrasound 2009;50(3):330–5.
25. Gieger T, Haney S, Nolan MW. Re-irradiation of canine non-lymphomatous nasal tumors using stereotactic radiation therapy (10 Gy x 3) for both courses: assess-ment of outcome and toxicity in 11 dogs. Vet Comp Oncol 2022;20(2):502–8.
26. Reczynska AI, LaRue SM, Boss MK, et al. Outcome of stereotactic body radiation for treatment of nasal and nasopharyngeal lymphoma in 32 cats. J Vet Intern Med 2022;36(2):733–42.
27. Yoshikawa H, Gieger TL, Saba CF, et al. Retrospective evaluation of intranasal carcinomas in cats treated with external-beam radiotherapy: 42 cases. J Vet Intern Med 2021;35(2):1018–30.
28. Swan MB, Morrow DM, Lurie DM. Pilot study evaluating stereotactic body radia-tion therapy for feline facial squamous cell carcinomas. J Feline Med Surg 2021; 23(12):1081–8.
29. Gualtieri P, Martin T, Leary D, et al. Canine salivary gland carcinoma treated with stereotactic body radiation therapy: a retrospective case series. Front Vet Sci 2023;10:1202265.
30. Lee BI, LaRue SM, Seguin B, et al. Safety and efficacy of stereotactic body radi-ation therapy (SBRT) for the treatment of canine thyroid carcinoma. Vet Comp On-col 2020;18(4):843–53.
31. Kelsey KL, Kubicek LN, Bacon NJ, et al. Neuromuscular blockade and inspiratory breath hold during stereotactic body radiation therapy for treatment of heart base tumors in four dogs. J Am Vet Med Assoc 2017;250(2):199–204.
32. Magestro LM, Gieger TL, Nolan MW. Stereotactic body radiation therapy for heart-base tumors in six dogs. J Vet Cardiol 2018;20(3):186–97.
33. Kruckman-Gatesy CR, Ames MK, Griffin LR, et al. A retrospective analysis of ste-reotactic body radiation therapy for canine heart base tumors: 26 cases. J Vet Cardiol 2020;27:62–77.
34. Trageser E, Martin T, Hoaglund E, et al. Outcomes of dogs with thymoma treated with intensity modulated stereotactic body radiation therapy or non-modulated hypofractionated radiation therapy. Vet Comp Oncol 2022;20(2):491–501.
35. Dolera M, Malfassi L, Pavesi S, et al. Volumetric-modulated arc stereotactic radio-therapy for canine adrenocortical tumours with vascular invasion. J Small Anim Pract 2016;57(12):710–7.
36. Linder T, Wakamatsu C, Jacovino J, et al. Stereotactic body radiation therapy as an alternative to adrenalectomy for the treatment of pheochromocytomas in 8 dogs. Vet Comp Oncol 2023;21(1):45–53.

37. Swan M, Morrow D, Grace M, et al. Pilot study evaluating the feasibility of stereotactic body radiation therapy for canine anal sac adenocarcinomas. Vet Radiol Ultrasound 2021;62(5):621–9.

38. King CR, Brooks JD, Gill H, et al. Long-term outcomes from a prospective trial of stereotactic body radiotherapy for low-risk prostate cancer. Int J Radiat Oncol Biol Phys 2012;82(2):877–82.

39. Nolan MW, Marolf AJ, Ehrhart EJ, et al. Pudendal nerve and internal pudendal artery damage may contribute to radiation-induced erectile dysfunction. Int J Radiat Oncol Biol Phys 2015;91(4):796–806.

40. Langberg CW, Waldron JA, Baker ML, et al. Significance of overall treatment time for the development of radiation-induced intestinal complications. an experimental study in the rat. Cancer 1994;73(10):2663–8.

41. Fitzpatrick CL, Farese JP, Milner RJ, et al. Intrinsic radiosensitivity and repair of sublethal radiation-induced damage in canine osteosarcoma cell lines. Am J Vet Res 2008;69(9):1197–202.

42. Farese JP, Milner R, Thompson MS, et al. Stereotactic radiosurgery for treatment of osteosarcomas involving the distal portions of the limbs in dogs. J Am Vet Med Assoc 2004;225(10):1567–72, 1548.

43. Martin TW, Griffin L, Custis J, et al. Outcome and prognosis for canine appendicular osteosarcoma treated with stereotactic body radiation therapy in 123 dogs. Vet Comp Oncol 2021;19(2):284–94.

44. Kubicek L, Vanderhart D, Wirth K, et al. Association between computed tomographic characteristics and fractures following stereotactic radiosurgery in dogs with appendicular osteosarcoma. Vet Radiol Ultrasound 2016;57(3):321–30.

45. Nolan MW, Green NA, DiVito EM, et al. Impact of radiation dose and pre-treatment pain levels on survival in dogs undergoing radiotherapy with or without chemotherapy for presumed extremity osteosarcoma. Vet Comp Oncol 2020; 18(4):538–47.

46. Boston SE, Vinayak A, Lu X, et al. Outcome and complications in dogs with appendicular primary bone tumors treated with stereotactic radiotherapy and concurrent surgical stabilization. Vet Surg 2017;46(6):829–37.

47. Martin TW, LaRue SM, Griffin L. CT characteristics and proposed scoring scheme are predictive of pathologic fracture in dogs with appendicular osteosarcoma treated with stereotactic body radiation therapy. Vet Radiol Ultrasound 2022; 63(1):82–90.

48. Swift KE, LaRue SM. Outcome of 9 dogs treated with stereotactic radiation therapy for primary or metastatic vertebral osteosarcoma. Vet Comp Oncol 2018; 16(1):E152–8.

49. Medin PM, Foster RD, van der Kogel AJ, et al. Spinal cord tolerance to single-session uniform irradiation in pigs: implications for a dose-volume effect. Radiother Oncol 2013;106(1):101–5.

50. Benedict SH, Yenice KM, Followill D, et al. Stereotactic body radiation therapy: the report of AAPM Task Group 101. Med Phys 2010;37(8):4078–101.

51. Rancilio NJ, Bentley RT, Plantenga JP, et al. Safety and feasibility of stereotactic radiotherapy using computed portal radiography for canine intracranial tumors. Vet Radiol Ultrasound 2018;59(2):212–20.

52. Klein EE, Hanley J, Bayouth J, et al. Task Group 142 report: quality assurance of medical accelerators. Med Phys 2009;36(9):4197–212.

53. Nolan MW, Randall EK, LaRue SM, et al. Accuracy of CT and MRI for contouring the feline optic apparatus for radiation therapy planning. Vet Radiol Ultrasound 2013;54(5):560–6.

54. Ericksen T, Mauldin N, Dickinson R, et al. Single high-dose radiation therapy and liquid fiducial markers can be used in dogs with incompletely resected soft tissue sarcomas. J Am Vet Med Assoc 2023;261(10):1–8.
55. Gieger TL, Nolan MW. Treatment outcomes and target delineation utilizing CT and MRI in 13 dogs treated with a uniform stereotactic radiation therapy protocol (16 Gy single fraction) for pituitary masses: (2014-2017). Vet Comp Oncol 2021;19(1):17–24.
56. Hansen KS, Zwingenberger AL, Théon AP, et al. Long-term survival with stereotactic radiotherapy for imaging-diagnosed pituitary tumors in dogs. Vet Radiol Ultrasound 2019;60(2):219–32.
57. Kent MS, Bommarito D, Feldman E, et al. Survival, neurologic response, and prognostic factors in dogs with pituitary masses treated with radiation therapy and untreated dogs. J Vet Intern Med 2007;21(5):1027–33.
58. Gieger T, Nolan M, Magestro L, et al. Stereotactic radiation therapy (SRT) versus full-course, fractionated radiation therapy (FRT) for canine pituitary masses: a comparison of protocols. American College of Veterinary Radiology Annual Forum; 2021.
59. Lawrence J, Forrest L, Adams W, et al. Four-fraction radiation therapy for macroscopic soft tissue sarcomas in 16 dogs. J Am Anim Hosp Assoc 2008;44(3):100–8.
60. Cancedda S, Marconato L, Meier V, et al. Hypofractionated radiotherapy for macrocroscopic canine soft tissue sarcoma: a retrospective study of 50 cases treated with a 5 x 6 Gy protocol with or without metronomic chemotherapy. Vet Radiol Ultrasound 2016;57(1):75–83.
61. Gagnon J, Mayer MN, Belosowsky T, et al. Stereotactic body radiation therapy for treatment of soft tissue sarcomas in 35 dogs. J Am Vet Med Assoc 2020;256(1):102–10.
62. Tierce R, Martin T, Hughes KL, et al. Response of Canine Soft Tissue Sarcoma to Stereotactic Body Radiotherapy. Radiat Res 2021;196(6):587–601.
63. Hansen KS, Li CF, Théon AP, et al. Stereotactic radiotherapy outcomes for intraventricular brain tumours in 11 dogs. Vet Comp Oncol 2023;21(4):665–72.
64. Carter GL, Ogilvie GK, Mohammadian LA, et al. CyberKnife stereotactic radiotherapy for treatment of primary intracranial tumors in dogs. J Vet Intern Med 2021;35(3):1480–6.
65. Moirano SJ, Dewey CW, Haney S, et al. Efficacy of frameless stereotactic radiotherapy for the treatment of presumptive canine intracranial gliomas: a retrospective analysis (2014-2017). Vet Comp Oncol 2020;18(4):528–37.
66. Swift KE, McGrath S, Nolan MW, et al. Clinical and imaging findings, treatments, and outcomes in 27 dogs with imaging diagnosed trigeminal nerve sheath tumors: a multi-center study. Vet Radiol Ultrasound 2017;58(6):679–89.
67. Dolera M, Malfassi L, Marcarini S, et al. High dose hypofractionated frameless volumetric modulated arc radiotherapy is a feasible method for treating canine trigeminal nerve sheath tumors. Vet Radiol Ultrasound 2018;59(5):624–31.
68. Hansen KS, Zwingenberger AL, Theon AP, et al. Treatment of MRI-diagnosed trigeminal peripheral nerve sheath tumors by stereotactic radiotherapy in dogs. J Vet Intern Med 2016;30(4):1112–20.
69. Dolera M, Malfassi L, Bianchi C, et al. Frameless stereotactic radiotherapy alone and combined with temozolomide for presumed canine gliomas. Vet Comp Oncol 2018;16(1):90–101.
70. Dolera M, Malfassi L, Pavesi S, et al. Stereotactic volume modulated arc radiotherapy in canine meningiomas: imaging-based and clinical neurological posttreatment evaluation. J Am Anim Hosp Assoc 2018;54(2):77–84.

Updates in Surgical Oncology

Bernard Séguin, DVM, MS, DACVS-SA, DECVSq[a],*,
Julius M. Liptak, BVSc, MVetClinStud, FANZCVc, DAVCS[b]

KEYWORDS

- Partial limb amputation • Prosthesis • 3D-printing • Limb sparing • Mast cell tumor
- Proportional margins • Grade shifting

KEY POINTS

- Partial limb amputation with a prosthesis is possible in dogs but complications are common.
- Double amputation is reported in dogs and cats and can lead to a good quality of life but more needs to be learned before it can be recommended broadly.
- Three-dimensional printing has been used for limb sparing in dogs but complications are still common.
- The recommendation for removing mast cell tumors in dogs is to perform a proportional margin excision.
- With the recurrence of a canine mast cell tumor or soft tissue sarcoma, grade shifting may have occurred.

New data and knowledge in small animal medicine and surgery have been acquired in recent years that have changed the approach to certain neoplasms or may change how we address certain neoplasms in the future. Here, we present selected updates in veterinary surgical oncology: new concepts regarding amputations, new developments for limb sparing, and new recommendations for the resection of cutaneous mast cell tumors (MCTs).

ADDRESSING TUMORS AFFECTING THE LIMBS: AMPUTATION AND LIMB SPARING
Partial Limb Amputation and Use of a Prosthesis

The most common treatment of dogs and cats with primary bone tumors, such as osteosarcoma, to address the local tumor is amputation. Amputation can also be a treatment of tumors of the soft tissues, such as MCTs and soft tissue sarcomas

[a] Central Victoria Veterinary Hospital, 760 Roderick Street, Victoria, British Columbia V8X 2R3, Canada; [b] Capital City Specialty & Emergency Animal Hospital, 747 Silver Seven Road, Kanata, Ontario K2V 0A2, Canada
* Corresponding author.
E-mail address: bernard.seguin@VCA.com

Vet Clin Small Anim 54 (2024) 577–589
https://doi.org/10.1016/j.cvsm.2023.12.010
0195-5616/24/© 2023 Elsevier Inc. All rights reserved.
vetsmall.theclinics.com

(STSs), in the limb where a curative-intent surgery is the goal. Still, a complete excision is impossible without an amputation.

Full limb amputation has been the standard of care in dogs and cats, whereas partial limb amputation with the use of a prosthesis is standard practice in humans. A socket prosthesis has been used in dogs with a partial limb amputation.[1–4] Although prostheses are commercially available for dogs, they are still in the early stages of research, development, and clinical applications. Anecdotally, some dogs use the limb with the prosthesis like a normal limb, and others refuse to bear weight on the limb when the prosthesis is applied. To better define the outcome and function of the use of prostheses in dogs and to start to understand the reasons for the variation in use, studies have been performed.

Owner satisfaction and perception of the quality of life for their dog wearing a prosthesis has been high. One study reported that 21 out of 24 dogs (87.5%) had the same improved quality of life as they did before using a prosthesis based on owners surveyed.[1] In another study, 10 out of 12 owners (83.3%) reported a good to excellent quality of life following prosthesis placement.[2] In a retrospective study of 47 dogs fitted with a socket prosthesis, 46 owners reported positive satisfaction.[3] Using a clinical assessment scoring system, 42 of 47 dogs were scored to have acceptable to full function, and 5 dogs had unacceptable clinical function. A 62% short-term and 19% long-term complication rates were reported. Skin sores were the most common short-term and long-term complication. Outcome scores and owner satisfaction significantly varied among dogs with different durations of prosthesis wear, with a trend toward better outcomes associated with longer prosthesis wear. In this retrospective study in dogs, there was no correlation between the level of the defect and either owner satisfaction or clinical outcome.[3] However, it is important to point out that the most proximal level of amputation was midradius for the forelimb and midtibia for the hind limb.[3]

In a prospective study of canine partial limb amputation with socket prostheses, 12 dogs were evaluated.[4] Ten dogs were treated with thoracic limb amputation and 2 with pelvic limb amputation. The level of amputation was midradial diaphysis, leaving 48% to 76% of the radius intact in 5 dogs: 1 at the proximal aspect of the distal radial metaphysis, 2 at the antebrachiocarpal joint; 1 at the midmetacarpus; 1 at the distal metacarpus for the thoracic limb; and 1 at the tarsometatarsal joint and 1 at the intertarsal joint for the pelvic limb. Ten of 12 patients experienced complications, and 19 were reported. Seven of the 12 patients experienced greater than one complication. Complications following prosthesis fitting included difficulty keeping the device on the limb (n = 5), pressure sores from the prosthetic devices (4), bursal formation at the distal residuum with bursitis (4), latent surgical site infections once the limb was healed (2), owner-reported aversion to the prosthesis (2), papular and pustular dermatitis (1), and pain secondary to nerve entrapment within surgically placed hemoclips (1). Pressure sores were limited to mild partial thickness abrasions or ulcers, which resolved with minor adjustments to the prosthetic liners, shells, or strapping systems. Of significant importance, all 5 patients who experienced difficulty maintaining the prosthetic device on the limb had amputations proximal to the carpus. Additional straps and harnesses were added to the devices for improved suspension. Even with additional harnessing, these 5 patients continued to spontaneously come out of their prosthetic devices to varying degrees, ranging from several times per walk to a few times per week during vigorous activity. One dog was unable to maintain the prosthetic device for more than a few steps, and therefore, prosthetic device use was discontinued. Objective gait analysis was performed in 11 of the 12 dogs in this study. The last gait data collected was performed at 200 ± 152 days postprosthesis fitting, and percent body weight distribution (%BWD) at that time point was 23.4% to 34.1% (mean = 25.8%) of weight-bearing on the affected limb of dogs with thoracic limb amputations, and 16.2% of weight-bearing on the affected limb of 1 dog with a pelvic limb amputation (the other dog with a pelvic limb amputation did not have objective gait analysis performed). The normal %BWD is 30% for the thoracic limb and 20% for the pelvic limb.[4] Owner satisfaction in this study was also high with 10 out of 11 who responded to the survey stating they were happy with the decision to pursue partial limb amputation.

Level of limb defect has been demonstrated in humans to significantly correlate with clinical outcomes.[5,6] It is unknown if the clinical outcome can be good if the level of amputation is more proximal than the midradius and midtibia in dogs. None of the dogs in the studies reported had an amputation more proximal than the antebrachium or midtibia.[1-4] There is some concern that an amputation more proximal than the midradius or midtibia leaves a residual limb (residuum) too short to allow fixation of a socket prosthesis. With a short residuum, the prosthesis can fall off easily and consequently requires additional means of fixation, such as straps around the body's trunk. All dogs that experienced difficulty maintaining the prosthetic device on the limb had amputations proximal to the carpus in the prospective study[4,] and the most common complication in one retrospective study[1] was the prosthetic slipping off the residuum, often occurring in 37.5% of the limbs. Moreover, as the residuum becomes shorter, the prosthesis becomes longer relative to the total length of the limb, and it becomes less of an element to help with ambulation and propulsion and more of a device to help maintain balance with less mechanical means for the animal to lift it off the ground and move it in the cranio-caudal plane. Much remains to be learned about prosthetics in small animals, including their design and the surgical technical details of partial limb amputation to decrease the risk of complications and improve functional outcomes.

Double Limb Amputations in Dogs and Cats

The results of a study on double limb amputations in dogs and cats are of interest to the surgical oncologist.[7] Although the situation where 2 limbs requiring amputation is uncommon in surgical oncology, this scenario can arise from time to time: either a dog or cat was already amputated for trauma and a tumor arises in a limb or 2 limbs are affected by a neoplasm, either simultaneously or separate points in time. The study reported on 14 dogs and 4 cats.[7] None of the animals in the study was ipsilateral double amputees. Twelve patients were bilateral pelvic limb amputees, 4 were bilateral thoracic limb amputees, and 2 were contralateral thoracic and pelvic limbs. Ten were full limb amputations for both limbs. Objective ambulatory function was not reported with the main aim of the study to report owner satisfaction. Of the 10 patients with bilateral full limb amputations, 1 owner was strongly dissatisfied, 2 were mildly satisfied, and 7 were very satisfied with the outcome. Owners of 10 of the 14 dogs included in the study reported a satisfaction score of very satisfied, 3 were mildly satisfied, and 1 was strongly dissatisfied. Owners of all 4 cats in this study were very satisfied with the outcome.[7]

Important to the pet's perceived function and quality of life by their owners, none of the patients in this study was fitted for prosthetics, although 3 patients (2 dogs and 1 cat) were noted to have a wheelchair available to them.[7] Although none of the partial amputation patients used external prosthetics, 4 of these 9 patients used their stumps for some measure of ambulation or balance.[7]

Of noteworthiness when considering these results may be the weight of the dogs included in this study. The mean, median, and range of body weights of the dogs were 14.6 kg, 11.6 kg, and 1.9 to 30 kg, respectively.[7] Osteosarcoma can be a neoplasm that affects 2 limbs, although uncommonly. Patients affected by osteosarcoma are typically large to giant breed dogs. In one of the largest studies on canine osteosarcoma with 324 dogs,[8] the median body weight was 38.8 kg with a range of 21.2 to 94.5 kg. The dogs in the double amputation study were considerably smaller. Another consideration is the age of the animal. Dogs in the double amputation study had a mean age of 3.7 years (median, 3.4; range, 0.2–8.3 years) and cats had a mean age of 1.4 years (median, 1 year; range, 1.0–2.5 years).[7] The most common reason for the double amputation in this study was trauma. By contrast, animals afflicted by cancer are generally older. For example, in the osteosarcoma study with 324 dogs, the median age was 8.1 years (range, 1.4–15.0).[8] The reason age may be an important factor is because of possible degenerative joint disease being present in the other limbs. Degenerative joint disease is more prevalent in older dogs and cats. Although large and giant breed dogs and dogs with some degenerative joint disease can still be excellent candidates for a single limb amputation, weight and the presence of degenerative joint disease may have a more important impact on the ability to adapt and function as a double amputee.

More data are required before double amputations can be recommended. Specifically, prognostic factors that would eventually evolve into candidature criteria need to be identified before this can become an accepted treatment option for dogs and cats.

Limb-Sparing Surgery

Limb sparing is a surgical option for some dogs with primary bone tumors where the tumor is removed but limb function is preserved. Some anatomic sites require reconstruction of the bone in some form. The scapula, distal ulna, metacarpal/metatarsal bones, and phalanx do not require reconstruction when the dog is a candidate for limb sparing.

The anatomic site most commonly reported for surgical limb sparing, and for which there are the most techniques described to reconstruct the bone, is the distal radius. The complication rate, however, remains high. In one study reporting on the technique using a metal endoprosthesis for reconstruction, 96% of dogs had a complication, and infection was the most common, with 78% of dogs being affected.[9]

Additive manufacturing, also known as three-dimensional (3D) printing, is a fabrication process that enables the design and manufacture of patient-specific prostheses, thus ensuring that the medical device can be perfectly adapted to the patient's morphology. For example, the radius can have a natural curvature in the mediolateral plane but that curvature is quite variable from one dog to another (**Fig. 1**). Commercially available implants are straight, and traditional plates cannot be bent in this plane. Therefore, they do not align well and do not allow a good fit between the limb-sparing plate and the proximal aspect of the radius (**Fig. 2**). With 3D printing, it is possible to create an implant that is the best fit for each dog (**Fig. 3**). Because the implant will be created to have the best fit and alignment, performing the osteotomy at the exact location it was intended and at the intended angle is crucial. For this reason, a cutting guide is also designed and printed to ensure the perfect osteotomy, and hence fit, for each dog (**Fig. 4**).

The workflow for 3D printing starts with a computed tomography (CT) of the limbs.[10] It is best to image the limb with the tumor and the contralateral limb, which will be used as a mirror image to help create the implant. Close communication between the surgeon and the engineering team designing and manufacturing the implant is paramount. Using the CT, the surgeon determines where the osteotomy in the radius will be positioned.

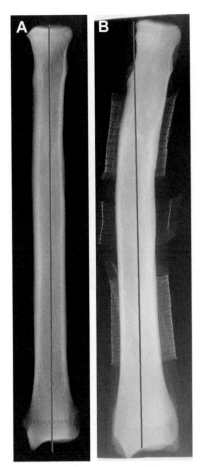

Fig. 1. Radiographs of 2 canine radii in the craniocaudal view. A red straight line has been placed in the center of the distal radius. The radiographs and lines demonstrate the variation that is possible in the curvature of the proximal radius in the mediolateral plane in dogs. The *red line* also dissects the radius in the center at the proximal aspect in A whereas the line is not even on the radius at the proximal aspect in B.

The next step is the reconstruction of the bones in silico.[10] The DICOM images are transferred to the engineering team. The images are processed using software (eg, Mimics Research19, Materialise, Leuven, Belgium), and the reconstructed bone structures will then be used for the implant and cutting guide designs. A segmentation procedure is finally carried out to separate the radius, ulna, and carpal/metacarpal bones on the affected limb and the healthy radius on the contralateral limb. The bone models are exported in stereolithography (STL) format into a computer-aided design environment.

The following step is the design of the titanium endoprosthesis and the cutting guide.[10] The bone model is converted from STL to solid, using software (eg, Catia V5R21, Dassault Systèmes, Vélizy-Villacoublay, France). The contralateral (healthy) radius, which is of similar size and proportion, is mirrored and superimposed on the affected radius. Next, the osteotomy plane is created at the prescribed distance perpendicular to the long axis of the bone. The affected part of the radius is virtually

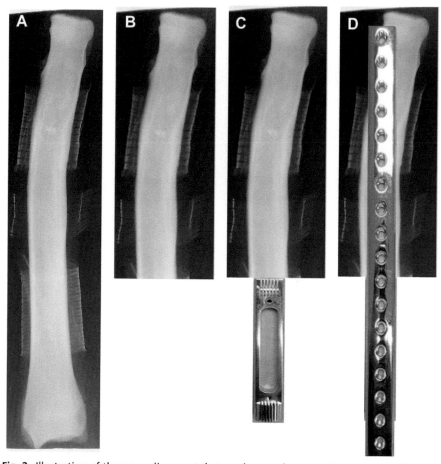

Fig. 2. Illustration of the poor alignment that can happen between the commercially available implants and the proximal aspect of the radius with limb sparing. (*A*) Radiograph of a canine radius in the craniocaudal view with a substantial curvature at its proximal aspect in the mediolateral plane. (*B*) Approximately 50% of the distal aspect has been "removed," as is the case with many limb-sparing cases for distal radial osteosarcoma. (*C*) A commercially available metal endoprosthesis has been placed in the defect to replace the distal aspect of the radius, such as is done with limb sparing. (*D*) A commercially available limb-sparing plate has been placed in alignment with the metal endoprosthesis (now covered by the plate and not visible). Because the plate is straight but the radius has a curvature, the alignment between the plate and the proximal aspect of the radius is poor.

removed and replaced by its healthy counterpart. A contoured plate, which can feature conical locking threaded holes, is created to accept commercially available screws. Afterward, the contoured plate, the healthy radius section, and an intramedullary stem, corresponding to 70% of the intramedullary canal diameter, are joined via additive Boolean operations. Then, subtractive Boolean operations are carried out to ensure perfect surface contact between the endoprosthesis and the bones: the carpal/metacarpal bones and the salvaged part of the affected radius are removed from the plate. Finally, the implant thickness is verified, and thin areas are reinforced. A parametric cutting guide template is placed on the radius and

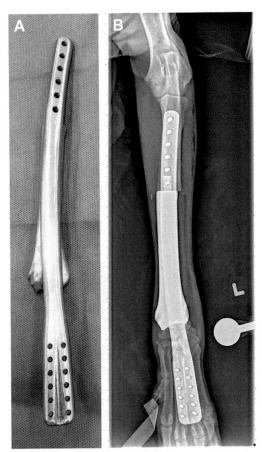

Fig. 3. (*A*) Picture of a personalized 3D-printed endoprosthesis showing the curvature in the mediolateral plane. (*B*) Postoperative radiograph in the craniocaudal view showing excellent alignment between the endoprosthesis and the radius.

adjusted to comply with the bone geometry. It features a cutting slot that coincides with the previously created osteotomy plane, ensuring correct alignment between the cut and the endoprosthesis. Before the manufacturing stage, the endoprosthesis and guide designs are validated with the veterinary surgeon and then converted into STL file format.

The next step in the workflow is manufacturing the endoprosthesis and cutting guide.[10] The endoprosthesis is manufactured using a Ti-6Al-4 V alloy powder (Ti64) and a laser powder bed fusion printer. During manufacturing, the endoprosthesis is oriented horizontally, thus reducing the build time and the amount of powder feedstock required, proportional to build height. After manufacturing, the build plate is cleaned of loose powder. The finishing and polishing steps follow this. The finished endoprosthesis is cleaned in an ultrasonic bath with a cleaning solvent. The cutting guide is fabricated from plastic, which can be acrylonitrile butadiene styrene plastic. The endoprosthesis and cutting guide kit are ready to be shipped to the veterinary clinic, where both must be sterilized before surgery.

The theoretic advantage of using 3D-printed personalized endoprostheses and cutting guides is that it may reduce the risk of some complications associated with other

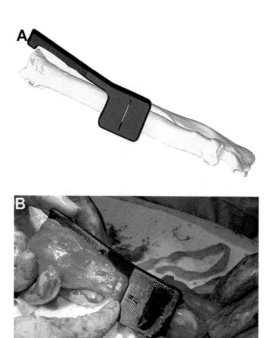

Fig. 4. (*A*) Computerized image showing the cutting guide hooked on the styloid process of the ulna and positioned on the radius. (*B*) Intraoperative image of the cutting guide in place for the radial osteotomy. The elbow is to the right and the manus has been disarticulated from the antebrachium. (Reprinted with permission from Seguin B, Pinard C, Lussier B, et al. Limb-sparing in dogs using patient-specific, three-dimensional-printed endoprosthesis for distal radial osteosarcoma: A pilot study. Vet Comp Oncol 2020;17:92–104.)

non–patient-specific limb-sparing surgical options. By having implants that align perfectly with the bones of the patient, the transfer of mechanical forces between the bones of the animal and implants when the limb bears weight should be optimal and consequently reduce the risk of biomechanical complications. Moreover, by having implants that fit perfectly onto the bones, there is no need for intraoperative bending of the implants, thereby reducing surgery and anesthesia times and the risk of infection.

One of the most significant disadvantages of using 3D-printed personalized implants for limb sparing is the time it takes for all of the steps previously involved, from performing the CT to the surgeon receiving the endoprosthesis and cutting guide. During this period, the tumor can continue to grow in size and affect how much bone should be removed. However, the endoprosthesis is designed with a specific, predetermined length of the bone to be removed. In one study using 3D-printed implants for reconstruction of the radius, tibia, or mandible after tumor removal, the size of the tumor progressed during the period between imaging and surgery thus requiring more extensive surgery in 25% of the dogs.[11] This had an impact on how the endoprosthesis was able to fit with the bones and led to complications in one dog.[11] Furthermore, incomplete surgical margins or local recurrence occurred in 33% of these dogs. In that particular study, the time interval between CT and surgery was not specifically reported but was up to 4 weeks. This demonstrates that delaying surgery is a serious and legitimate concern when using personalized, 3D-printed implants for reconstruction in oncologic surgery.

In a prospective study using 3D-printed personalized endoprostheses, the time interval between CT and surgery was 14 days,[12] which seemed reasonable to minimize the risk of excessive tumor growth in that interval; however, the engineering team thought this was not a realistic and achievable time frame for every dog. The engineering team expressed that every step had to be performed at maximum efficiency, without any incident, to allow this. It was unlikely that this was possible with every dog to be enrolled in the study. To provide more time to perform the reconstruction, design, and manufacturing of the personalized implant, intra-arterial (IA) chemotherapy was given at the time of CT to the other dogs enrolled in the study. IA chemotherapy using cisplatin in dogs has been shown to induce significant necrosis to appendicular OSA, whereas intravenous chemotherapy did not.[13,14] In the prospective study, carboplatin was administered IA instead of cisplatin.[12] The interval between CT and surgery in the dogs receiving IA carboplatin (n = 4) was 23 to 70 days. Three out of 4 dogs had the tumor decrease in size. The planned margins for the osteotomy were deemed adequate in all cases at the time of surgery and all achieved complete margins; however, 1 dog developed local recurrence 24 weeks postoperatively.[12] Local recurrence following complete histologic resection has been reported in 4% to 30% of dogs after limb-sparing surgery of the distal radius.[15–17]

Other postoperative complications in the prospective study included infection in all 5 dogs, biomechanical complications in 2 dogs, and complications with the skin in 2 dogs.[12] Using objective gait function analysis, the limb achieved near normal function but unsurprisingly complications negatively affected its function. Unfortunately, the results of small studies using 3D-printed endoprostheses and cutting guides so far did not have results to suggest that their use can decrease the risks of complications. More studies are needed to optimize the use of this approach and hopefully reap its biomechanical benefits.

One of the areas of limb-sparing surgery in dogs where 3D printing may provide a better solution is for the primary bone tumors involving the proximal humerus. Alternatives to limb amputation for proximal humeral tumors include intraoperative radiation therapy, stereotactic radiation therapy (SRT), or surgical limb sparing using an allograft. Intraoperative radiotherapy, reported in 5 dogs with proximal humeral osteosarcoma, led to complications in all dogs, including bone fracture, implant failure, infection, and radial nerve paralysis.[18] The most common major complication with SRT is fracture. More than 50% of dogs have a fracture at 11 months after SRT.[19,20] Using an allograft for the proximal humerus site has resulted in high complication rates and poor limb function.[21] There are, therefore, currently no viable options for preserving the limb for dogs with proximal humeral osteosarcoma with an acceptable risk of complications. Three-dimensional printing can allow the design and manufacturing of more complex endoprostheses for the shoulder joint, which may lead to improved function and decreased complications.

Studies have been done to understand the shoulder joint's complexity. Three different types of endoprostheses have been proposed: the monobloc endoprosthesis, which leads to arthrodesis of the shoulder joint; an endoprosthesis with a revolute joint, which allows motion only in the craniocaudal plane; and an endoprosthesis with a spherical joint, which allows motion in all planes. Identification of the muscles that are likely necessary to be preserved during the limb-sparing surgery to have a functional shoulder joint with each kind of endoprosthesis has been reported.[22,23]

Another possibility that 3D printing allows is the design and manufacturing of endoprostheses made of biodegradable and bioreplaceable materials. Specifically, endoprostheses made of β-tricalcium phosphate, with or without polycaprolactone, permit the replacement of the endoprosthesis with the growth of the host bone. One such endoprosthesis was used in an Akita for limb sparing of distal radial osteosarcoma.[24] On postoperative radiographs, some opacity developed in the endoprosthesis suggestive of bone regeneration. The dog died 190 days postoperatively, and a necropsy was not possible to determine the true extent of bone regeneration. In another case of distal radius limb-sparing surgery, but in this case, the distal diaphysis rather than metaphysis, a Yorkshire terrier had an atrophic nonunion, which led to a critical size defect.[25] The defect was filled with a 3D-printed β-tricalcium phosphate scaffold. Complete healing of the radius was noted radiographically 4 months after surgery, and the bone plate was removed 10 months after surgery.[25] The critical size defect had been completely replaced by the host bone. Although not a cancer case, this exemplifies the ability of these materials to allow host bone ingrowth. These 2 cases received recombinant human bone morphogenetic protein-2 (RhBMP-2) to promote bone healing and growth. Its use in cancer cases is controversial because it may promote the growth of cancer cells but may be necessary to allow full replacement of the scaffold by host bone. One dog with a parosteal osteosarcoma of the zygomatic arch had the tumor removed, and the zygomatic arch was replaced with a 3D-printed polycaprolactone/β-tricalcium phosphate scaffold. This dog did not receive RhBMP-2. At 10 months postoperatively, the scaffold was not entirely replaced by bone based on CT examination.[26] Once again, more research is needed to better define the optimal mixture of polycaprolactone and β-tricalcium phosphate for mechanical strength and bone ingrowth and the role of RhBMP-2 or any other agent that promotes bone growth on the risk of enhancing local recurrence of the neoplasm and its necessity for full bone ingrowth.

MAST CELL TUMOR

Historically, the recommendation for curative-intent resection of cutaneous MCTs was 2 to 3 cm lateral margins around the tumor and one uninvolved fascial plane deep to the tumor.[27] More recent evidence suggests that this is not necessary, and newer data support the recommendation to resect cutaneous MCTs with proportional margins. With this paradigm, the lateral margins are equivalent to the widest dimension of the MCT, with an upper limit of 2 to 4 cm, with the deep margin remaining an uninvolved fascial plane.[28–31] Using the proportional margin approach, 85% to 95% of tumors had complete histologic excision with a local recurrence rate of 0% to 3%. The histologic grade of the cancer (high vs low using the Kiupel grading scheme) was not prognostic for obtaining complete margins in one study.[30] In contrast, it was not possible to evaluate grade as a prognostic factor for completeness of excision in other studies.[28,29,31] Incomplete margins may be more likely with larger tumors (>10 mm; P=.06 in one study); however, local recurrence was independent of completeness of surgical excision.[30] Histologic grade is prognostic for local recurrence with local recurrence only reported or suspected in dogs with high-grade MCTs.[28,30] Other MCT studies not related to the investigation of proportional margins have also found that high-grade tumors were significantly more likely to have a local recurrence, demonstrating that histologic grade is an important prognostic factor for local recurrence.[32,33]

Grade Shifting

On the topic of local recurrence, the clinician should be aware that grade shifting is possible with local recurrence in dogs. Grade shifting is where the tumor at the time of local recurrence is of a different, usually higher, grade than when the first tumor was resected. Grade shifting was documented in 1 of 5 MCTs where the MCT was low grade initially and high grade at the time of recurrence.[34] Grade shifting was also reported in 7 of 15 dogs with STSs where the STS was higher grade in 4 tumors at the time of recurrence and lower grade in 3 tumors.[34]

CLINICS CARE POINTS

- When using a personalized implant that is 3D-printed for limb sparing, intra-arterial chemotherapy should be considered to prevent the tumor from growing excessively in the period betweem doing the CT to plan the prosthesis and performing the limb sparing surgery.
- When resecting cutaneous mast cell tumors in dogs, surgical margins should be based on the proportional margin paradigm.
- when local recurrence has occured with canine mast cell tumor or soft tissue sarcoma, clinical decisions should not be made based on the grade of the previous tumor removed as grade shifting might have occured.

DISCLOSURE

B. Séguin has no commercial or financial conflict of interest to disclose. J.M. Liptak is on the board of QBiotics Group.

REFERENCES

1. Carr BJ, Canapp S, Petrovitch JL, et al. Retrospective study on external canine limb prosthesis used in 24 patients. Vet Evid 2018;3:1.
2. Phillips A, Kulendra E, Bishop E, et al. Clinical outcome and complications of thoracic and pelvic limb stump and socket prostheses. Vet Comp Orthop Traumatol 2017;30:265–71.
3. Wendland TM, Seguin B, Duerr FM. Retrospective multi-center analysis of canine socket prostheses for partial limbs. Front Vet Sci 2019;6:100.
4. Wendland TM, Seguin B, Duerr FM. Prospective evaluation of canine partial limb amputation with socket prostheses. Vet Med Sci 2023;9:1521–33.
5. Esquenazi A. Amputation rehabilitation and prosthetic restoration. From surgery to community reintegration. Disab Rehabil 2004;26:831–6.
6. Treweek SP, Condie ME. Three measures of functional outcome for lower limb amputees: a retrospective review. Prosthet Orthot Int 1998;22:178–85.
7. Magidenko SR, Peterson NW, Pisano G, et al. Analysis of patient outcome and owner satisfaction with double limb amputations: 14 dogs and four cats. J Am Vet Med Assoc 2022;260:884–91.
8. LeBlanc AK, Mazcko CN, Cherukuri A, et al. Adjuvant sirolimus does not improve outcome in pet dogs receiving standard of care therapy for appendicular osteosarcoma: a prospective, randomized trial of 324 dogs. Clin Cancer Res 2021;27:3005–16.
9. Mitchell KE, Boston SE, Kung M, et al. Outcomes of limb-sparing surgery using two generations of metal endoprosthesis in 45 dogs with distal radial osteosarcoma. a veterinary society of surgical oncology retrospective study. Vet Surg 2016;45:36–43.

10. Timercan A, Brailovski V, Petit Y, et al. Personalized 3D-printed endoprostheses for limb sparing in dogs: Modeling and in vitro testing. Med Eng Phys 2019;71: 17–29.

11. Bray JP, Kersley A, Downing W, et al. Clinical outcomes of patient-specific porous titanium endoprostheses in dogs with tumors of the mandible, radius, or tibia: 12 cases (2013-2016). J Am Vet Med Assoc 2017;251:566–79.

12. Seguin B, Pinard C, Lussier B, et al. Limb-sparing in dogs using patient-specific, three-dimensional-printed endoprosthesis for distal radial osteosarcoma: A pilot study. Vet Comp Oncol 2020;17:92–104.

13. Withrow SJ, Thrall DE, Straw RC, et al. Intra-arterial cisplatin with or without radiation in limb-sparing for canine osteosarcoma. Cancer 1993;71:2484–90.

14. Powers BE, Withrow SJ, Thrall DE, et al. Percent tumor necrosis as a predictor of treatment response in canine osteosarcoma. Cancer 1991;67:126–34.

15. Seguin B, Walsh PJ, Ehrhart EJ, et al. Lateral manus translation for limb-sparing surgery in 18 dogs with distal radial osteosarcoma in dogs. Vet Surg 2018;48: 247–56.

16. Withrow SJ, Liptak JM, Straw RC, et al. Biodegradable cisplatin polymer in limb-sparing surgery for canine osteosarcoma. Ann Surg Oncol 2004;11: 705–13.

17. Séguin B, O'Donnell MD, Walsh PJ, et al. Long-term outcome of dogs treated with ulnar rollover transposition for limb-sparing of distal radial osteosarcoma: 27 limbs in 26 dogs. Vet Surg 2017;46:1017–24.

18. Liptak JM, Dernell WS, Lascelles BDX, et al. Intraoperative extracorporeal irradiation for limb sparing in 13 dogs. Vet Surg 2004;33:446–56.

19. Kubicek L, Vanderhart D, Wirth K, et al. Association between computed tomographic characteristics and fractures following stereotactic radiosurgery in dogs with appendicular osteosarcoma. Vet Radiol Ultrasound 2016;57: 321–30.

20. Martin TW, Griffin L, Custis J, et al. Outcome and prognosis for canine appendicular osteosarcoma treated with stereotactic body radiation therapy in 123 dogs. Vet Comp Oncol 2021;19:284–94.

21. Kuntz CA, Asselin TL, Dernell W, et al. Limb salvage surgery for osteosarcoma of the proximal humerus: outcome in 17 dogs. Vet Surg 1998;27:417–22.

22. Le Bras L-A, Timercan A, Llido M, et al. Personalized endoprostheses for the proximal humerus and scapulo-humeral joint in dogs: Biomechanical study of the muscles' contributions during locomotion. PLoS One 2022; 17(1):e0262863.

23. Llido M, Brailovski V, Le Bras L-A, et al. Muscular morphometric study of the canine shoulder for the design of 3D-printed endoprostheses in dogs with osteosarcoma of the proximal humerus: a pilot cadaveric study by MRI. J Am Vet Res 2023;84. ajvr.22.12.0220.

24. Choi S, Oh Y-I, Park K-H, et al. New clinical application of three-dimensional-printed polycaprolactone/β-tricalcium phosphate scaffold as an alternative to allograft bone for limb-sparing surgery in a dog with distal radial osteosarcoma. J Vet Med Sci 2019;81:434–9.

25. Franch J, Barba A, Rappe K, et al. Use of three-dimensionally printed β-tricalcium phosphate synthetic bone graft combined with recombinant human bone morphogenic protein-2 to treat a severe radial atrophic nonunion in a Yorkshire terrier. Vet Surg 2020;49:1626–31.

26. Kyu-Won K, Jin-Hyung S, Hyun-Jung K, et al. Zygomatic arch reconstruction with a patient-specific polycaprolactone/beta-tricalcium phosphate scaffold after parosteal osteosarcoma resection in a dog. Vet Surg 2022;51:1319–25.

27. Thamm DH, Vail DM. Mast cell tumors. In: Withrow SJ, Vail DM, editors. Small animal clinical oncology. 4th edition. St Louis: Saunders Elsevier; 2007. p. 402–24.

28. Pratschke KM, Atherton MJ, Sillito JA, et al. Evaluation of a modified proportional margins approach for surgical resection of mast cell tumors in dogs: 40 cases (2008–2012). J Am Vet Med Assoc 2013;243:1436–41.

29. Chu ML, Hayes GM, Henry JG, et al. Comparison of lateral surgical margins of up to two centimeters with margins of three centimeters for achieving tumor-free histologic margins following excision of grade I or II cutaneous mast cell tumors in dogs. J Am Vet Med Assoc 2020;256:567–72.

30. Saunders H, Thomson MJ, O'Connell K, et al. Evaluation of a modified proportional margin approach for complete surgical excision of canine cutaneous mast cell tumours and its associated clinical outcome. Vet Comp Oncol 2020; 19:604–15.

31. Itoh T, Kojimoto A, Uchida K, et al. Long-term postsurgical outcomes of mast cell tumors resected with a margin proportional to the tumor diameter in 23 dogs. J Vet Med Sci 2021;83:230–3.

32. Donnelly L, Mullin C, Blako J, et al. Evaluation of histological grade and histologically tumour-free margins as predictors of local recurrence in completely excised canine mast cell tumours. Vet Comp Oncol 2015;13:70–6.

33. Kry KL, Boston SE. Additional local therapy with primary re-excision or radiation therapy improves survival and local control after incomplete or close surgical excision of mast cell tumors in dogs. Vet Surg 2014;43:182–9.

34. Griffin MA, Hughes K, Altwal J, et al. Grade shifts in recurrent canine soft tissue sarcomas and mast cell tumors. J Am Vet Med Assoc 2023;261:1–8.

A Practical Guide to Clinical Studies in Veterinary Oncology

Kristen Weishaar, DVM, MS[a],*, Kai-Biu Shiu, BVMS, MRCVS[b],
Zachary M. Wright, DVM[c]

KEYWORDS

- Clinical trials • Clinical studies • Oncology • Veterinary medicine • Private practice
- Audits • Adverse events

KEY POINTS

- Recognize the practicalities, benefits, and challenges associated with developing a clinical studies program.
- Understand the infrastructure needed to successfully participate in clinical studies in academic and private practice settings.
- Understand the financial and regulatory implications of clinical studies.
- Recognize the expectations for data management, adverse event reporting, and on-site audits.

COMMON ABBREVIATIONS AND DEFINITIONS USED IN CLINICAL STUDIES

Acronym		Definition
AE	Adverse event	An unfavorable or unintended clinical finding noted after initiation of a study
ALCOA	Attributable, legible, contemporaneous and accurate	Guidance for how study data are recorded
BED	Biologically effective dose	Dose needed to cause expected biologic effect of drug
CRF	Case report form	Documents used to capture all study data during visits
		(continued on next page)

[a] Colorado State University Flint Animal Cancer Center, CSU Veterinary Teaching Hospital, 300 West Drake Road, Fort Collins, CO 80523, USA; [b] VCA VESVSC, 1612 North High Point Road, Middleton, WI 53562, USA; [c] VCA Animal Diagnostic Clinic, 4444 Trinity Mills Suite 100, Dallas, TX 75287, USA
* Corresponding author.
E-mail address: Kristen.Weishaar@colostate.edu

Vet Clin Small Anim 54 (2024) 591–601
https://doi.org/10.1016/j.cvsm.2023.12.011
0195-5616/24/© 2023 Elsevier Inc. All rights reserved.

vetsmall.theclinics.com

(continued)		
Acronym		**Definition**
CRO	Contract research organization	A hired third party that manages a study for a sponsor and serves as the point of contact for study sites
DLT	Dose-limiting toxicity	Side effect that is severe enough to discontinue treatment at that dose
EDC	Electronic data capture	Platform for digitally recorded and stored CRFs
GCP	Good Clinical Practice	Industry standard for conduct of clinical studies including data collection and documentation
IACUC	Institutional Animal Care and Use Committee	Regulatory body to ensure appropriate and ethical animal treatment during studies
IIS	Investigator initiated study	Clinical study designed and conducted by an investigator at an institution
IRB	Institutional review board	A group of experts that reviews the detailed plan of a clinical study for scientific quality and correct study design
IVP	Investigational veterinary product	The product in question for a study evaluation
MTD	Maximally tolerated dose	Highest dose of drug or treatment that can be given without unacceptable side effects
SAE	Serious adverse event	Adverse event that is life threatening or could result in long-term disability. Important to differentiate from a severe AE, which refers to the intensity of the adverse event; an AE may be considered severe based on grade but of minor medical significance
SOP	Standard operating procedure	Standardization document designed to ensure procedures are performed consistently and correctly
VCSC	Veterinary Clinical Studies Committee	Committee that serves to ensure that research is conducted in accordance with ethical standards; convened when studies fall outside the purview of an IACUC

INTRODUCTION

Research creates the foundation on which clinical decisions in veterinary oncology are based. Specialist training requires critical evaluation of the medical literature to understand the impact of study design on the study's findings. Many trainees have the opportunity to design or participate in clinical studies through their residency training programs because many academic institutions have established oncology clinical study teams or departments.

The goal of this article is to describe the opportunities, perspectives, and considerations for pursuing clinical studies beyond a training program in both private practice and academic settings. The infrastructure needed to effectively implement clinical studies will also be discussed. There are minimal peer-reviewed publications on these topics; as such, the majority of the content in this article is based on the authors' personal experiences with clinical studies in both private practice and academic settings.

INCORPORATING CLINICAL STUDIES INTO AN ONCOLOGY SERVICE: BENEFITS AND CHALLENGES

Clinical studies have several benefits to an oncology service. They may challenge an oncologist intellectually with new procedures, therapies, or diagnostics, which can provide variety and an element of job satisfaction. On an individual level, participation in studies may contribute to a feeling of being part of something bigger, thus contributing to job satisfaction and reducing burnout. Clinical studies can widen access to cancer therapy for clients that cannot afford standard treatments. Additionally, clinical studies often supersede commercial availability by 3 to 5 years. Thus, participation in clinical studies accelerates the learning curve for diagnostics or therapeutics that successfully reach the market. Clients participating in studies often appreciate the altruistic aspect of their pet contributing to medical advances, potentially helping future animals and people with cancer.

Clinical studies can provide a diversified revenue stream. Generally, there is direct compensation from a sponsor for conducting the study and data collection. Indirect revenue may exist from ancillary services including surgery, imaging, and hospitalization. Finally, there may be a bystander effect of increased patient referrals to the practice with intent for enrollment in a clinical study. Referrals may grow based on the knowledge that an institution has a reputable and active portfolio of clinical studies.

Conversely, conducting clinical studies is costly and time consuming, with requirements for specific/additional infrastructure, equipment, and qualified personnel. Documentation and clinical study processes such as informed consent and following Good Clinical Practice (GCP) guidelines are significantly more time consuming than standard practice and can quickly escalate exponentially as subjects are enrolled.[1] The importance of anticipating the time burden associated with clinical study paperwork and responding to sponsor/monitor queries cannot be underestimated, particularly when developing a budget with a clinical study sponsor.

Participating as an investigator in a clinical study (with an approved protocol and schedules) can be constraining for a clinician that is used to responding instinctively to unexpected findings or adverse events (AEs). Seeking approval from principal investigators or sponsors for individual cases and situations can add a layer of delay, frustration, and uncertainty for the investigator and client. Even the most minor deviations from a study protocol will require additional paperwork and written explanations.

Clinical Studies in Private Practice

With thought and commitment, developing a clinical studies program within a busy private specialty practice is an achievable goal.

In the authors' opinion, a successful clinical study program requires a large team effort. The scenario that is most likely to prove unsuccessful is a single clinician who has interest in studies trying to participate by themselves. All doctors in a specific department should be committed to participating in the study, as scheduling proves problematic when only a single doctor can meet the enrollment needs. Additionally, patient accrual is much more successful when all doctors are willing to have the same prestudy enrollment discussions with potential participants.

The technical staff should also be both encouraged to participate in studies and rewarded for their efforts. Reminding the technical staff that this is a form of career development that makes them more marketable in the future has proven to be a successful strategy in the author's hospital. Monetary incentive may be an additional driver of participation for support staff.

There are several mechanisms for a clinician to fund or participate in a clinical study. The majority of clinical studies in private practice are industry-sponsored, although nonprofit foundations such as the Morris Animal Foundation and others have competitive processes for awarding research funding. Larger corporations (Blue Pearl, VCA, MedVet, and so forth) have clinical studies departments that are designed to recruit sponsors and negotiate contract details before implementation at the clinic level. For clinicians in those facilities, alerting their specific studies division to your interest is generally all that is required. There may also be opportunities to serve as a study site for clinical studies that originate from academic institutions or through contract research organizations. Self-designed clinical studies are not recommended as an initial starting point due to the complexity and steep learning curve. For those in an independent private practice environment, the authors recommend taking the time to establish some basic infrastructure (GCP training, and so forth) and then pursue word of mouth networking opportunities to highlight your interest and capabilities to sponsors.

Once training and infrastructure have been finalized, your team is ready to participate. The authors suggest participating in low-demand studies (ie, simple sample collection) to start. These studies usually only require noninvasive sampling and minimal paper record keeping. It allows the practice to establish a workflow with paperwork, recheck scheduling, and so forth and improves the staff's comfort level in discussing client consent forms.

As a clinical study progresses, the staff's learning curve will obviously improve. In the author's practice, this generally means slow accrual rates for the first 3 to 5 cases and then a steep linear increase in accrual through the remainder of the study.

Clinical Studies in Academia

The existing infrastructure and support services that are often present in an academic setting can make the initiation and conduct of veterinary clinical studies more straightforward but include their own set of challenges and potential roadblocks.

Clinical studies in academia generally fall into 2 broad categories: investigator-initiated studies (IISs) and industry-sponsored studies. An IIS is a clinical study designed by an investigator who has proposed a research topic and is responsible for creating the study protocol, whereas industry-sponsored studies are conceived of by an outside organization, such as a pharmaceutical company, and implemented at research sites. In general, IISs aim to answer questions that are more clinically relevant and provide results that can be applied to a more generalized patient population.[2] However, there are challenges associated with conducting IISs, in that many of the tasks that are the responsibility of the sponsor and their staff in industry-sponsored studies fall onto the investigator. These include protocol design, data management, and statistical analysis, among others. Finances also tend to be a significant barrier in IISs because study activities are limited by the amount of funding the investigator receives.

Externally funded research at academic institutions is generally managed by a group called Sponsored Programs. These individuals are involved in all steps needed to initiate a research project at the institution, including review of proposals and budgets before submission, contract negotiations, and administration of funds received. The oversight provided by this group can be very beneficial in removing these responsibilities from the investigator's purview but can also add a significant amount of time to the process, depending on staffing and workload.

Several veterinary academic institutions have a centralized clinical studies core, which provides support to investigators throughout the hospital in the conduct of their clinical studies. These groups are composed of veterinarians, technicians, co-ordinators, and other support staff who specialize in clinical research. Tasks that may be performed in the prestudy setting include assistance with grant and budget development, interaction with Sponsored Programs, submission for regulatory (ie, IACUC) approval, and case report form (CRF) design. Once the clinical study is un-derway, these individuals can assist in patient recruitment, study coordination, obtaining informed consent, data management, and study monitoring. They are also often directly involved with patient visits for studies, including providing tech-nical support, sample collection and processing, and data documentation. All of these services are provided at a cost to the investigator and therefore must be built into the budget in advance. At institutions without a clinical studies center, the inves-tigator and their support staff generally manage these tasks. Depending on the num-ber of investigators and active clinical studies, a service within the hospital may have specific staff dedicated to clinical studies, including technicians and a clinical studies coordinator.

INFRASTRUCTURE DEVELOPMENT AND STAFF TRAINING

Once a hospital is committed to clinical study participation, a basic infrastructure should be established before cases are enrolled. Key members of a clinical research team include the Principal Investigator (PI), study clinicians, technicians, and a study coordinator. The PI is the person who oversees all aspects of a research study and is responsible for reviewing, analyzing, and reporting data collected in the study. This person may or may not be the one who initially conceived of the study aims and design. The study clinicians are the doctors who provide medical care for the patients enrolled in the study. Technicians are responsible for sample collections, treatment administrations, routine medical care, data capture, and client communications. The study coordinator supports and facilitates daily study activities to ensure the protocol is being followed. This person may also be involved in patient recruitment and obtain-ing informed consent. In some instances, a study technician may also serve as the coordinator. In human medicine, each study generally has its own specific research team. In veterinary medicine, these individuals are often involved in multiple clinical studies within a service or hospital. Updated Curriculum Vitae for all participating staff should be kept on file by the study coordinator because they are generally required for all clinical studies.

Along with veterinarians and their immediate technician support staff, there may be other individuals within a hospital who play an active role in study management. This may include client service representatives, pharmacy staff members, and designated laboratory technicians or shipping "experts." All these individuals should be included in study participation and training.

Training for clinical studies staff members should include basic instruction in the completion of CRFs, including documentation of AEs and concomitant medications. In addition, team members should understand the importance of following all proto-cols and standard operating procedures (SOPs) specific to a study, as well as report-ing of protocol deviations, serious AEs, and Notes to File. GCP training is also essential to a successful clinical study program. GCP is an internationally accepted standard for clinical study participation that covers safety, medical ethics, and study record keep-ing to ensure study data integrity.[1] GCP training may be provided internally by the hos-pital or veterinary company, by a study sponsor, or through an external third party. Finding group training time within the workday is often a more successful model than individual self-directed learning.

For more advanced studies (blinded, pivotal, and so forth), sponsors will usually initiate both a site visit and training session for all participants. All individuals who will play a role in the conduct of the study should attend these training sessions, including clinical research team members, pharmacy staff, and client service representatives. Only individuals trained on the study are generally allowed to participate in the study. This means that data collected by nontrained employees may be tainted and censored. Be prepared that these training sessions generally require several hours for completion.

EQUIPMENT AND FACILITY NEEDS

Clinical studies require some physical plant specifications, although these may vary depending on the complexity of the studies that are conducted at a certain site. Ample storage space, such as cabinets or shelving units, is needed for regulatory and patient binders as well as study-specific clinical supplies. Securing documents with a locking mechanism is preferred. Depending on a hospital's workflow and information technology (IT) capabilities, designated computers or laptops for clinical study work may prove useful. Various office supplies, such as a copier, document scanner, and 3-hole punch are also needed. For clinics with a national IT ecosystem, it is important to eliminate various website blockers to allow for access to necessary training sites and CRF programs. DICOM viewers should have a mechanism to export and share imaging outside of the electronic medical record (EMR). Additionally, internal cloud sharing allows for ease of data transfer from electronic medical records to study CRFs.

Additional supplies and equipment will be necessary for clinical studies that require collection and processing of samples for study purposes, such as blood and tumor tissue. These may include centrifuges, pipettes, cryovials, blood collection tubes with various and unique substrates, access to a biosafety cabinet and/or fume hood, a liquid nitrogen supply, and refrigerators and freezers (-20°C, -80°C) for sample storage. Calibration, certification, and monitoring of weighing scales and refrigeration may be required.

DATA MANAGEMENT

Data management is the process of collection and management of data in a clinical study in accordance with the study protocol and regulatory standards.[3,4] It is a critical part of clinical research because it leads to the generation of high-quality, reliable, and statistically sound data. The ultimate goal is to ensure that the conclusions drawn from research are well supported by data. Specific guidelines for data management are provided in the GCP regulations and the US Food and Drug Administration (FDA) guidance document 21 CFR Part 11.[1,5]

There are several steps involved in data management, which begin during clinical study development and continue throughout the course of the study and beyond.[3,4] Design of data collection instruments (ie, CRFs) is a key first step to ensure that data collected are complete and accurate. These forms should be concise, self-explanatory, user-friendly, and collect data in a manner that allows for the most efficient and consistent extraction.[6] A general guiding principle to ensure data integrity is that all data collected should be attributable, legible, contemporaneous, and accurate. A common phrase used in reference to data collection in clinical studies is as follows: "If it is not documented, then it did not happen."

CRFs may be paper or electronic/web-based, and there are several online data capture systems available for use in veterinary clinical studies at various price points. Several features of electronic CRFs allow added assurance of data integrity over paper forms, including having control over the ability to alter previously entered data, providing an audit trail and time stamps for changes to data, protection from data tampering, and safe storage of data. Electronic data capture also allows for remote data monitoring, facilitates collaborations among institutions, and streamlines the extraction of data for analysis.

Data validation is an ongoing review of subject data that occurs throughout the duration of a clinical study. The goal of this process is to confirm that the data documented in CRFs are accurate and complete, and correlate with the information in patient medical records. Data must be verified and reported according to the study protocol, any SOPs, and regulatory guidelines. Data validation may be performed by the investigator or other study staff members, or by a Clinical Research Monitor appointed by the study sponsor. Any data found to be incorrect or missing must be amended. For clinical studies with a designated monitor, study sites should expect to schedule time for periodic on-site evaluations and intermittent calls with the sponsors. These meetings generally only require the primary investigator and study coordinator's participation. As the study progresses, sponsors will begin to closely analyze the data and provide feedback (queries). For an inexperienced staff, queries can be an overwhelming time commitment of which additional financial compensation is generally not provided. It is recommended that participants remember their GCP training and use more diligence at the onset of record keeping to prevent debilitating query buildup.

ADVERSE EVENT REPORTING

An adverse event (as defined by GCP guidelines), is any unfavorable or unintended sign (including an abnormal laboratory finding), symptom, or disease temporally associated with the use of an investigational product (IP), whether or not it is thought to be related to the IP.[1] Documentation of AEs that occur throughout the course of a clinical study is an important step in the assessment of the risks associated with the intervention under investigation.

AEs can be identified through multiple avenues, including review of the history or journals provided by a pet owner, physical examination findings, and assessment of diagnostics performed at a visit. Any finding that was not present at the baseline evaluation, or has increased in severity since baseline evaluation, should be documented as an AE. The dates of onset and resolution and treatment required must also be recorded.

Once an AE has been identified, it must be assessed for severity, attribution, and expectedness. Severity of AEs in veterinary oncology studies is assigned using the Veterinary Cooperative Oncology Group—Common Terminology Criteria for Adverse Events (VCOG-CTCAE).[7] This document allows for standardization of AE reporting across groups/sites and clinical studies. AEs are grouped into broad categories (ie, Gastrointestinal, Metabolic/Laboratory), and each AE is listed individually with criteria for grading on a scale of 1 to 5, based on severity. It is recommended that multiple copies of the VCOG-CTCAE be placed throughout a facility for ease of access.

Attribution of an AE is an evaluation of what the event may be related to and the likelihood of the relation. Possible attributions may include the IP, the existing neoplasia, underlying concurrent medical conditions, a procedure performed as part of the study, or another cause. Assigning an attribution in oncology clinical studies can be particularly challenging because clinical study protocols are often complex and involve multimodality therapy. Patients often have multiple symptoms and signs present at the time of enrollment into the study and are often on concurrent medications that may affect the occurrence and/or severity of AEs. Some questions to consider when assigning attribution of an AE are as follows:

- What are the known side effects of the study intervention?
- What is the temporal relationship of the AE to the study therapy?
- Does the AE improve or resolve when treatment is stopped?
- Does the AE reappear when study treatment is resumed?
- How does the AE relate to signs/symptoms of the existing cancer, abnormalities observed at baseline, or underlying medical conditions?

It is important to identify not only to what the AE is related but also to what it is not related. The relationship to each possible attribution (ie, IP, existing neoplasia, concurrent medical condition, study procedure, and so forth) should be assigned as unrelated, unlikely, possible, probable, or definite. These attributions can help determine what steps should be taken to treat the individual patient, as well as make decisions about protocol modifications that may be necessary to prevent similar AEs in other patients.

AEs are also classified as either expected or unexpected. An AE is considered unexpected if it is not listed as a possible side effect in study-related documents, including informed consent. An expected AE that occurs at a higher grade than what has previously been reported can also be considered unexpected.

An AE may be classified as serious (serious adverse event [SAE]) if any of the following apply.

- Results in patient death
- Is life threatening
- Requires hospitalization (initial or prolonged)
- Results in disability or permanent damage
- Causes a congenital anomaly/birth defect
- Requires intervention to prevent permanent impairment/damage
- Other serious events that do not fit into other categories

A study protocol should have specific criteria as to what constitutes an SAE for that particular study. Any grade 4 or 5 AE is generally considered an SAE. For clinical studies using chemotherapy agents, grade 3 nonhematologic AEs are usually classified as SAEs, whereas grade 3 hematologic AEs are not because these tend to be self-resolving and not associated with other significant complications. SAEs also have specific reporting requirements, which should be outlined in the study protocol. In general, these should be reported to the PI/sponsor within 24 hours, and also need to be reported to any regulatory bodies (ie, IACUC) in a timely fashion. If the study is a pivotal study for FDA approval, then all SAEs must be reported to the FDA.

AUDITING

Any site that participates in an FDA-approved or USDA-approved study may be subject to an external audit. Auditors will first call to speak with the primary site investigator to alert the study site to the audit. A facility is generally given 7 to 10 days to accommodate the request. Walk-in audits with no warning are possible.

If an audit has been triggered, a facility should immediately contact the study sponsor and monitor. A quality sponsor should provide an audit SOP. The facility will designate a private workspace and a host for the auditor to ensure their needs are met and that the auditor is only given access to the facility and data they require.

Consider the following recommendations for an audit visit.

1. Ensure the study binder is up to date with the latest version of the protocol and appendices
2. Ensure the drug accountability trail is complete and accurate
3. Remove all unnecessary materials and signage from the facility. Examples of this include bulletin board postings intended to provide hospital levity, and so forth
4. Ensure all participating staff is available to meet with the auditor if needed
5. Be engaged, honest, and present during one-on-one time with the auditor
6. Answer questions as succinctly as possible to prevent triggering additional questions with a long-winded answer
7. Provide the auditor with any additional documentation that is requested
8. Do not provide any documents related to the study that are not requested, or information on other clinical studies
9. Do not allow the auditor to tour the facility unsupervised
10. Do not offer the auditor food or beverages because this can be considered coercion

FINANCIAL IMPLICATIONS OF CLINICAL STUDIES

The degree of funding for a clinical study will vary according to the intensity and study design. Some studies will provide a financial incentive to the owner (rebate or payment toward standard therapy), some studies are fully funded (no cost to owner), and some may simply cover the cost of a therapeutic and/or potential adverse effects.

When considering the financial implications from the clinical investigator's perspective, discussion of indirect costs (to cover overheads such as facilities, equipment use and maintenance, employment benefits, computing/office equipment, and management) will not be discussed in detail here because these are often published costs not directly related to a specific project but the research institution as a whole. These will be set by the institution but may be negotiable and generally are a set percentage. Indirect costs usually do not apply to private practices because the cost of overheads generally is accounted for with existing pricing. However, in both settings, the additional time and skills required for implementing a clinical study should be captured in some manner.

Direct costs are those directly connected to the specific study, including clinical costs, salaries, wages, benefits, materials and supplies, equipment, and travel expenses. In academic settings, certain clinical costs may be provided at a discounted rate for patients enrolled in clinical studies to allow funds budgeted for IISs to be maximally used.

The time associated with training should be specifically budgeted. The data collection requirements associated with each visit should be financially captured independent of routine medical services. As a reminder, there is a high likelihood of additional data management following review of source information by monitors. This is especially important for clinical studies that are conducted according to GCP standards. GCP requires real-time data collection so study appointments generally are scheduled in longer intervals. Additionally, most studies require more frequent visitation schedules and testing than what is generally recommended in routine disease management. Prestudy workflow should also include mechanisms for determining who was involved (doctor and staff) at each study visit. The per hour cost of staff time can be roughly estimated by collating the average hourly rates of investigators and support staff involved.

Study-related remuneration of staff and clinicians will vary among institutions. A hospital's payroll department should be consulted before sponsorship agreements to ensure that the funds are allocated appropriately.

REGULATORY OVERSIGHT OF CLINICAL STUDIES

Clinical studies in academia are generally regulated by an Institutional Animal Care and Use Committee (IACUC), which is responsible for the oversight of all research involving animals at an institution, including clinical studies. PIs are responsible for providing specific information about study protocols to the IACUC, and the committee must approve the protocol before any research activities can begin. An IACUC can also suspend research projects at any time. The committee also inspects facilities where research is performed. Because the IACUC is generally more familiar with regulations for research in laboratory animals, some veterinary academic institutions also use a clinical review board, which specializes in review of clinical studies using client-owned animals.

In the private practice setting, larger corporate entities may house their own internal committee for review of study protocols. The American Veterinary Medical Association (AVMA) has published guidance on the establishment of Veterinary Clinical Studies Committees to serve this purpose.[8] A recent article from the AVMA Council on Research provides suggested best practices for scientific and ethical review of veterinary clinical research studies and supplements the guidance provided by the AVMA.[9] Alternatively, private practices may rely on a sponsor's internal IACUC or an academic institution's IACUC when collaborating in larger multisite studies.

SUMMARY

Participating in clinical studies can be rewarding, interesting, and fulfilling; the experience can also be frustrating, tedious, and time consuming. Training, diligence, and development of good processes throughout the organization will set the team up for success.

CLINICS CARE POINTS

- Participating in clinical studies can be intellectually rewarding and provide an added level of job satisfaction. However, challenges exist in the need for specific infrastructure and training, as well as the time constraints placed on clinic staff.
- Commitment of the entire clinic team is vital to the success of a clinical studies program.
- All staff participating in clinical studies should be trained in GCP and be vigilant in following the guidelines.
- Data management and validation are key steps in the conduct of clinical studies, and dedicated time must be allowed for these tasks.
- Accurate and complete documentation of AEs, including severity, attribution, and expectedness is required to fully assess the risks associated with an investigational treatment.

DISCLOSURE

The authors have no conflicts of interest to declare.

REFERENCES

1. International Council for Harmonisation of Technical Requirements for Pharmaceuticals for Human Use (ICH). Integrated addendum to ICH E6(R1): guideline for good clinical practice E6(R2). Step 4 version dated 9 November 2016. Available

at: https://database.ich.org/sites/default/files/E6_R2_Addendum.pdf. Accessed August 8, 2023.

2. Konwar M, Bose D, Gogtay NJ, et al. Investigator-initiated studies: Challenges and solutions. Perspect Clin Res 2018;9(4):179–83.

3. Krishnankutty B, Bellary S, Kumar NB, et al. Data management in clinical research: An overview. Indian J Pharmacol 2012;44(2):168–72.

4. Matkar S, Gangawane A. An outline of data management in clinical research. Int J Clin Trials 2017;4(1):1–6.

5. FDA Guidance Document Part 11, Electronic Records; Electronic Signatures - Scope and Application. Available at: https://www.fda.gov/regulatory-information/search-fda-guidance-documents/part-11-electronic-records-electronic-signatures-scope-and-application. Accessed August 8, 2023.

6. Bellary S, Krishnankutty B, Latha MS. Basics of case report form designing in clinical research. Perspect Clin Res 2014;5(4):159–66.

7. LeBlanc AK, Atherton M, Timothy Bentley R, et al. Veterinary Cooperative Oncology Group-Common Terminology Criteria for Adverse Events (VCOG-CTCAE v2) following investigational therapy in dogs and cats. Vet Comp Oncol 2021;19(2):311–52.

8. American Veterinary Medical Association Policy: Establishment and use of veterinary clinical studies committees. Available at: https://www.avma.org/resources-tools/avma-policies/establishment-and-use-veterinary-clinical-studies-committees. Accessed October 9, 2023.

9. Baneux PJR, Bertout JA, Middleton JR, et al. Perspectives on implementing veterinary clinical studies committees. J Am Vet Med Assoc 2023;261(9):1–6.

Moving?

Make sure your subscription moves with you!

To notify us of your new address, find your **Clinics Account Number** (located on your mailing label above your name), and contact customer service at:

Email: journalscustomerservice-usa@elsevier.com

800-654-2452 (subscribers in the U.S. & Canada)
314-447-8871 (subscribers outside of the U.S. & Canada)

Fax number: 314-447-8029

Elsevier Health Sciences Division
Subscription Customer Service
3251 Riverport Lane
Maryland Heights, MO 63043

*To ensure uninterrupted delivery of your subscription, please notify us at least 4 weeks in advance of move.